The Dukan Diet 100 Eat As Much As You Want Foods

By Pierre Dukan

With the invaluable help of
Carole Kitzinger and Rachel Levy

HODDER &
STOUGHTON

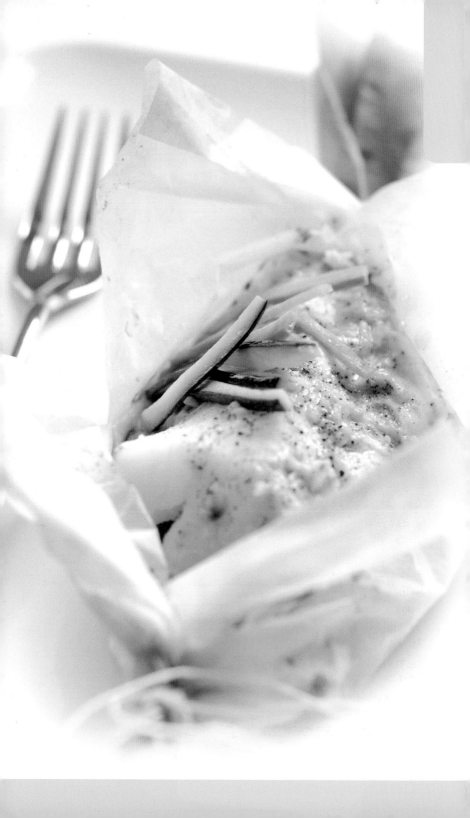

Contents

Poultry

Fish

Seafood

Eggs

Dairy Products

Vegetable Proteins

Vegetables

Sauces

Introduction

Once war has been declared and you are preparing to enter the fray, your best counsel is to start off by checking your weapons and munitions, your maps and provisions.

Losing weight is a war – one that is unusual and occasionally rewarding, as you have to do battle with yourself. I have learnt from over 30 years of experience on this battlefield that the greatest enemies in the struggle to lose weight are the pacifists, those people who think that in order to tackle the dangers and violence of weight problems all that is needed is common-sense advice and appeals to reason and equilibrium. As the Barbarians were laying siege to Byzantium, the clerical elite were busy debating whether angels were male or female; yet all around them the Huns and Alans were demolishing the gates to their city! 'Eat less, exercise more' is just pious hope when you are not given the ways and means to make this happen.

Returning to my war and to the method that uses the 100 foods described in this book: I need to present them in their proper context.

You may perhaps think that in using such martial vocabulary I am overdramatizing what is a simple matter of being overweight. You would be sorely mistaken, because what might have been a 'simple matter' 15 years ago has today turned into nothing less than a serial killer that is possibly more harmful than Aids and swine flu combined. And this is without taking into account the collateral damage, the economic cost and the suffering inflicted on those people who are transformed by their weight problems to such an extent that they no longer recognize themselves.

So if I talk about warfare it's because this is indeed a war and the fact that you have bought this book makes me think that you are well aware of this. I know how helpless you feel, because for over 30 years I have been listening to you confide in me about it. Moreover, it is because I am a doctor and have watched you suffer while feeling helpless myself that I devised my method, by trial and error, by constantly making improvements, by listening to your questions, your personal experiences and your suggestions.

Today my method is complete, coherent, structured and comprehensive; everything that you tell me in your letters, emails and in face-to-face consultations leads me to believe that this method is ready to go and confront the dragon's gaping jaws and take on this global weight epidemic that nothing so far has managed to prevent from marching onwards into conquered land.

For this method of warfare, I have drawn up a battle plan that includes phases and stages and successive campaigns, a target which is Each Individual's True Weight, a flag and victories, but one which also allows for wintertime trenches and immobility, setbacks and lapses. And one day the final battle will result in a victory with an armistice based on a negotiated weight. The treaty will be signed but with an enemy that bides its time, eager to take up arms again to recapture its lost spoils. Then everything will pass into the hands of the people and it is they who will have to defend this peace, they who will have to learn what the risks are and how to protect themselves from these dangers. This war has often been waged but without peace ever being established and, without peace, nothing is truly accomplished or gained.

Dear reader, perhaps you bought this book because you have heard about me or rather you know about my method; or perhaps you were simply attracted by the title. So, I am going to explain, in just a few pages, what lies behind these foods: a whole programme that has been put together over the years, over the decades, a programme that enables anyone who wants to lose weight to achieve their goal.

Think of these 100 foods as a quiver of arrows that you are going to carry with you as you head off to confront your surplus pounds – and you will certainly need them, of that you can be assured! Take heed: the 100 foods make complete sense only when used as part of my method, which allows you to eat them without any restriction as regards quantities, combinations or timing – just like a buffet! Before we take a closer look at these 100 foods, I will devote a few pages to setting out the main ideas behind my method.

The bedrock and principles of the Dukan Diet, and how to follow the method

The method, which my public decided to name after me, is my lifetime's work. Since becoming a doctor, initially working as a general practitioner, I have derived tremendous pleasure from treating anyone who could be helped. When I became a nutritionist, I tried to apply what I had been taught but very quickly I realized that if we used these particular tools we were fighting a losing battle. So, very early on, I created a diet,then a programme and then a method. At first, I did this for my patients, then for my readers, then for internet users and lastly for doctors, my medical colleagues. The whole programme came together like a community that has gradually crossed borders and cultures.

Today, with 35 years' experience and hindsight, I am firmly convinced that I can offer the very best way of putting up resistance to the weight-problem epidemic sweeping across the planet.

This method is based on six key concepts:
- **100 foods, 72 animal and plant proteins and 28 vegetables.**
- **You are allowed to eat AS MUCH AS YOU WANT of these 100 foods!**
- **A strong structure with four successive phases takes care of the person who wants to lose weight from the very first day and then forever more.**
- **Absolute top priority is given to consolidating and then permanently stabilizing your True Weight.**
- **Physical exercise is prescribed 'like medication on a prescription' and the top priority is WALKING.**
- **You are monitored through daily internet coaching that is personalized with TO instructions in the morning and a FRO report in the evening.**

My method has been devised to be a COMPLETE WHOLE. Each one of its stages has a particular purpose and cannot be carried out in isolation from the three other phases. So you have to follow it in its entirety or not embark on it at all. And, most important, you must follow the two stabilization phases, without which the whole enterprise will be doomed to failure.

In return, when adhered to as a whole, the diet offers you definite advantages and your motivation levels will remain unswerving for three reasons:

- The method gives you a list of very precise instructions, providing a strong framework that limits any constraints, wavering and frustration.
- The method offers you a completely natural diet. And of all natural diets it is the one that gets you the best results.
- Lastly, this diet is not frustrating; no restrictions regarding quantities are laid down.

Here I will set out the main principles behind my method and give you an overview to help you understand how to use it. However, if you feel in tune with this diet and the motivation to follow it, may I suggest that you invest a few pounds and buy a paperback copy of my book *The Dukan Diet* or *The Dukan Diet Life Plan*. These will help you understand how the method works, provide you with a complete road map and answer all the questions that anyone trying to lose weight might want to ask.

Furthermore, if you think that you need help, monitoring and support on a daily basis; if each morning you would like to receive your own instructions about what to eat and how to exercise along with some motivational support; if each evening you would like to send in your results so they can be analyzed to form the basis of new instructions to be sent to you the following day, you will find this help available on **www.dukandiet.co.uk**. You should enter the special code '100foods' to benefit from the special offer extended to my readers.

The Dukan Diet's four main phases

Phase 1: the Attack phase – pure proteins (PP)
This phase is based on 72 foods, including those with the highest protein content. It gets off to a lightning-quick start; weight loss is very rapid and highly motivating.

Phase 2: the Cruise phase – proteins with vegetables (PV)
The Attack period is followed by the Cruise phase, during which you will add 28 vegetables to the 72 high-protein foods, alternating between one day of proteins with vegetables and one day without vegetables until you get down to your True Weight.

Phase 3: the Consolidation phase

Once you have attained your True Weight, you must at all costs avoid the weight rebound phenomenon, which is when the body cannot help trying to put back on the pounds it has just lost. Be careful, as this phase is strategic and lasts five days for every pound lost.

Phase 4: the permanent Stabilization phase

Here you go back to eating what you want but with three simple, concrete, effective but non-negotiable measures to protect you; and, as your safety back-up, you have all the foods from the Consolidation phase.

The Attack phase

This is the period of greatest motivation as you watch the numbers on your scales drop at breathtaking speed – it is almost as if you were fasting but while eating AS MUCH AS YOU WANT.

This Attack programme is a real war machine. Your objective during this very brief phase is to feed yourself with some of the most natural foods you could possibly eat, foods that have been selected because they have the highest protein content, while ignoring the other nutrients. In reality, it is impossible to eliminate carbohydrates and fats from your diet totally. In fact, apart from egg white, there is no food that contains only protein. So your diet will bring together a certain number of foods that contain as much protein as possible with as little fat and carbohydrate as possible. These foods include some meats, fish, seafood, poultry (without the skin), eggs, cooked sliced meats (without any fat or rind) and fat-free dairy products.

Length of time: Depending on the individual, the circumstances and how much weight has to be lost, this period may last between two and seven days.

Results: For those with fewer than 10 pounds to lose, a couple of pounds may be shed in an Attack phase lasting two days; for those with 4–6 stone to lose, it may last one week with 7–11 pounds being shed. For the seriously obese, the Attack phase may last ten days.

The Cruise phase

The Cruise phase is when you alternate between pure proteins (PP) and proteins with vegetables (PV).

This second phase follows on from the Attack and introduces vegetables in patterns that can alternate to fit with different circumstances, gender, age and desired weight loss. However, the simplest way of alternating is to have one PP day followed by one PV day and so on. Just as with the Attack, the Cruise phase allows you the same complete freedom to eat the quantities you want, at the times you want and in whatever combination you want. These two successive phases are the equivalent of a buffet: you can eat all you like from it but anything that is not part of the buffet is not for you and you must forget all about it until you get down to your True Weight. The driving force behind the method is this lack of restriction combined with steady weight loss which means you will lose weight but will be shielded from feeling hungry and frustrated. These foods provide a base which will be yours to use for the rest of your life.

Length of time: You have to follow this phase without stopping until you attain the weight you are aiming for; weight loss amounts on average to a couple of pounds a week.

The Consolidation phase
Foods are reintroduced in two phases.

Like the three other phases, this one has its own particular job to do. It has been devised to act as a transition between all-out dieting and not dieting at all. Moving from one to the other is crucial and has to be handled very carefully. Enough foods have to be reintroduced to reward the dieter who has just attained their True Weight while avoiding the risk of any weight regain – in other words, the common and devastating 'rebound effect'.

Having been forced to lose weight, your body is going to make the most of this new-found freedom to eat other foods and it will try to regain some weight. The more weight it has shed, the more energy it will put into regaining those lost pounds.

It has two ways of doing this: it can drastically reduce the energy it burns up and it can increase its energy intake by extracting every last calorie from the food you eat. A copious meal that would have had little impact before embarking on a diet will now, during this Consolidation period, have serious repercussions. This is why quantities of over-rich foods must still be avoided while you wait for your metabolism to calm down and for this rebound effect to run its course, as this is the reason why weight-loss diets so often fail.

Length of time: This will depend on how many pounds have been lost and can be worked out very easily: five days for every pound lost.

For example, if you have lost ten pounds, you will spend 50 days in Consolidation; five pounds and it will be 25 days.

Along with the 100 protein foods and cruise vegetables you now add one then two pieces of fruit, two slices of wholemeal bread, 40g (1½oz) of cheese, one then two portions of starchy foods per week and one then two celebration meals per week. You continue with your pure-protein Thursdays to protect what you have achieved.

The Stabilization phase
Three simple measures for always.

Anyone who has followed a diet and lost weight knows full well, from having learnt at their own expense, that losing weight does not in itself provide any guarantee that the new weight you have attained will be stabilized and maintained. Quite the opposite: any dieting gives your body time and opportunity to learn how to resist dieting.

It is vital, therefore, that the weight you have consolidated continues to be kept under control, that you watch out for warning signs and retaliate with a series of graded counterattacks if any pounds do go back on. However, it is just as important that this control is sufficiently flexible and unobtrusive, so that you are happy to exercise it over the long term.

Three simple, concrete, easy and not-too-frustrating but non-negotiable measures offer you this control:

- Pure-protein Thursdays
- Giving up lifts and escalators + a 20-minute walk daily
- Three tablespoons of oat bran every day

Length of time: For as long as possible; even better, for the rest of your life – so that you can eat just like everyone else but without putting any weight back on.

Oat bran

This foodstuff is of course one of my 100 foods but it is far, far more than that – it is one of my method's foundations. It is the only foodstuff in the world that can claim to help you actually lose weight. Why? Oat bran has two physical properties which mean that as soon as it enters the digestive tract it turns into a sticky, viscous sponge whose beneficial qualities help you lose weight.

Absorption: The soluble fibre in oat bran is able to absorb on average up to 30 times its volume of water. Once it reaches the stomach, one 12g tablespoon will soak up 300g of water and will form a 312g ball that has enough volume to make you feel full very quickly and then satisfied over a long period.

Viscosity: Completely mixed in with all your other foods, the oat bran reaches the small intestine. At this point the food is a rich and nutritious pulp that is ready to pass into the bloodstream. This is when oat bran performs its main role. Since it is extremely viscous, the bran sticks to everything surrounding it, capturing and trapping the nutrients with which it comes into contact along with the calories in these nutrients and, as the bran cannot be absorbed, it takes them away with it as it is eliminated from the body in the stools. This way calories are lost, a modest amount to be sure, but this process can be repeated again and again and over a long period of time.

Furthermore, in addition to helping with weight problems, oat bran slows down the rate at which sugars are absorbed into the blood, it reduces cholesterol and helps keep bowel movements regular. Pure magic!

Oat bran is an integral part of my method. I prescribe it in doses that vary with each phase and it is included in my programme as follows:

- One and a half tablespoons per day in the Attack phase
- Two tablespoons per day in the Cruise phase
- Two and a half tablespoons per day in the Consolidation phase
- Three tablespoons per day in the Stabilization phase

Oat bran can be bought in health-food shops and supermarkets, and can be used to make galettes, pancakes, muffins, porridge and so on. You should be aware, however, that not all types of oat bran produce the same results. (To find out more, visit: **www.allaboutoatbran.com.**)

Most types of oat bran available today are manufactured according to traditional methods and are for cooking use only, so they are not always the most suitable if your aim is to stay slim and healthy. The bran's medicinal properties depend essentially on how it is milled and sifted. The milling determines to what extent the bran is ground and the size of its particles. Bran that has been over-milled is too fine; it is easier to cook with but it will have lost most of its slimming and health properties. Bran that is too coarse loses its viscosity and its ability to sneak away those calories. Sifting separates the oat flour, full of sugar, from the oat bran, which has little sugar but lots of fibre and proteins. Bran that has not been sufficiently sifted contains too much sugar; it is sweeter but less slimming.

In Finland, Europe's leading oat-bran producer, I have personally worked alongside agricultural engineers to marry clinical and biological data with production techniques. By working together we were able to come up with an index that establishes the very best nutritional properties for oat bran, and it combines an average M2 milling with B6 sifting. For the time being, these improvements mean that manufacturing costs are slightly higher, but if European producers were to join forces, the cost of culinary bran and nutritional bran could be standardized.

Taking exercise

If you are aiming to lose weight, taking exercise is not just necessary; it is absolutely essential! I have given up simply advising patients to take exercise – I now 'prescribe' it, just as I would prescribe medication. Surprisingly enough, prescribing exercise instead of merely recommending it has changed everything and the instruction is followed.

Being active has therefore become the second driving force behind my method and I call it PE: Prescribed Exercise.

Walking as weight-loss medication: Of all the forms of exercise available, I have decided to advocate walking. Why walking? Because it is the most natural, most effective, most inexpensive and most therapeutic activity there is. You can go walking anywhere and at any time, whatever you are wearing. It is also the only risk-free activity an obese person can undertake, however much they weigh.

You should walk at a regular pace and without interruption, breathing in deeply. Taking in sufficient oxygen is a tool that is overlooked in the weight battle. Always bear in mind that the body's metabolism needs oxygen to burn up stored fats efficiently.

The walking I prescribe as part of my programme is:

- 20 minutes per day in the Attack phase
- 30 minutes per day in the Cruise phase
- 25 minutes per day in the Consolidation phase
- 20 minutes per day in the Stabilization phase

In the Cruise phase, the dieter is inevitably beset by what I call 'plateaux', periods when weight loss slows down or stagnates – the main reason why diets fail or are abandoned. If this happens, increase your walking to one hour a day over four days to 'break through the plateau'.

Making physical activity a natural part of your daily routine: Apart from walking, I heartily recommend that you make the most of every opportunity in your daily life to use your body to perform useful tasks so that it gets accustomed to 'real life' again.

An army of robots has conspired to eradicate physical activity from our daily lives, along with all the gadgets that paralyze our activity, so try to wrest back from them your physicality – your body is half of what you are. I am not just philosophizing here, because in your case we are waging open warfare against your surplus pounds.

So give up taking lifts and escalators; if you have a dog, take it out for a good long walk; do your washing-up yourself; make your bed; do the vacuuming and work in the garden. Rediscover what your body, with its 800 muscles, was made for. The fact that those muscles are there, the sheer number of them and the way they are so deeply connected with the brain, proves that they are a crucially important part of human life. And that not using them as we are meant to can only result in 'punishment' being meted out.

Finally, try to adopt a different way of looking at your actions and movements. Concentrate on seeing any exertion not as some tedious, unwelcome and pointless effort but rather as an activity or movement with a meaning and purpose that will do you good. So if you drop something and it falls to the ground, instead of grumbling, pick it up with the most expansive movement possible, bending your knees rather than your back. This may appear a trivial example to you, but I can assure you that thinking about every simple movement you make will completely reverse the order of things at the very heart of the problem.

A major tool for the method – online, daily and personalized monitoring

True Weight: Losing weight and not putting it back on is a far more difficult and complex undertaking than it may appear. To get down to your True Weight, you really have to want to change, you need real motivation, and, for those who have many pounds to lose, you need a good diet. However, for the weight you attain to be maintained in the future, you will need something else too. Since dieters have often confused an attainable weight with a maintainable weight, they manage to lose weight but in a way that depressingly leads to weight regain.

If you are trying to lose weight over the long term, and to be cured of your weight problems, you need to know the weight you are able to attain and maintain. Each individual has a weight that they can achieve and at the same time hope to keep, and this will be based on gender, age, family background and heredity, bone structure, number of pregnancies, past history and battle against weight gain and the number of diets already tried. I have named this weight Each Individual's True Weight. To work it out, go to my website www.dukandiet.co.uk and answer the 11 questions you will be asked; you will then be given your reference weight. The calculation costs nothing. Knowing this weight is not just for curiosity's sake; it is highly strategic knowledge since it defines a point of reference and a norm calculated according to medical criteria. Knowing your True Weight means you will not set off to fight for some unrealistic goal or, worse, a target weight that shifts as you lose weight, or – worse still – a weight that you cannot possibly maintain and that will doom you to certain failure.

Monitoring and coaching on the internet

Almost two million readers have bought my book *The Dukan Diet*, which contains all the main information about my method and how to follow it. Of those who have read the book, I do not know how many have then followed my diet, or how many have reached their True Weight or, even less, how many have stabilized their weight permanently after completing the four phases.

However, I do know, from the many letters and emails I receive, that a good proportion of readers have managed to slim and stabilize the weight they got down to but also that some stopped after losing weight and did not go through the final two phases, the Consolidation and Stabilization phases, putting back on most of the weight they lost.

Then there are other people who have told me that they understood the method perfectly well and had kept to the spirit of it but that they did not have the strength to go the whole way on their own. To get there, they felt they needed to be accompanied, guided, supervised and supported, day after day, pound after pound.

I have always known this, because for me this support has become the essence of my work. Every day I see just how hard it is to give up eating and the easy way it gets you through all the ordeals, dissatisfactions and stresses of modern life, at work as well as socially and emotionally.

For those men and women, suffering from being overweight without being able to put it right, I searched for a solution and a way of supporting them that was personalized but could also be applied on a large scale, since in France there are only just over 300 doctors specializing in nutrition to deal with a clinically overweight population of 20 million people. In its time, I considered the supervision and monitoring offered by Weight Watchers as revolutionary. Having group meetings was such a good idea that it made up for the Weight Watchers' diet itself, based as it is on the old-fashioned system of calorie-counting. Nowadays, the explosion of new technologies and the ease of online communication means you do not have to travel and attend meetings in person to share your results and private thoughts.

So I decided to adapt my method to personalized monitoring on the internet.

At the time I made this decision, in France – and even more so in the USA – there were already websites that offered coaching for people with weight problems. I therefore took a look at them; as a medical professional, I tested and analyzed them to draw inspiration from the way they were set up. I was surprised to see that not one of them, not even the main American sites listed on the stock exchange, was offering a personalized relationship with the subscriber and, even less, any proper monitoring. Not one of them took, or even today takes, any account of what essentially defines coaching: the personality of its subscribers and the monitoring of their progress – none of the sites received any daily feedback from subscribers about their results or performance so that new instructions for the following day could be sent out.

A real weight-loss coach must be able to say to the person they are supporting and monitoring: 'I know you, I know who you are, why you have put on weight, and I am going to tell you, day after day, what you have to do to lose weight. And for your part of the deal, you will tell me how closely you have followed my instructions, so that tomorrow I can put you back on track and give you ways of putting things right or send you my congratulations to keep you motivated.'

Having seen that there was a huge gap here, I decided to set up a website that would offer this interactive personalization and monitoring: www.regimedukan.com – the original French site that was gradually rolled out to other countries and set up in different languages. Four years earlier, I had gained some expertise in this field when, with 32 volunteer doctors and a team of artificial intelligence engineers, we created the 'My Weight Book' project. With answers to 154 questions we had all the specific information about a particular individual to enable us to print uniquely for this person, and this person alone, a book that was posted directly to them (find out more at www.livredemonpoids.com).

I drew upon this experience to set up my own coaching website with a profiling system based on 24 questions and a patented communication process: the Daily To and Fro Email. This system meant that complete instructions could be sent out every morning without fail and every evening the subscriber could send back a report giving their weight, details of any lapses, any exercise undertaken, their motivation and frustration levels. Without knowing all this information, any coaching is unimaginable. Unfortunately, if you sign up to any other coaching website in any country today, whether you are male or female, a young teenage boy or a menopausal woman, a sporty person or someone who leads a sedentary lifestyle and smokes like a trooper, you will all receive exactly the same message with exactly the same instructions and nobody will ever know whether in fact you followed your instructions or not.

Through my international organization of nutritionists, RIPOSTE, I have been advocating that a service of this kind should be set up and I have offered to share my technology. I have personally put this proposal forward to the European health commissioner and I do hope that one day it will happen as there are already 1.3 billion people in our world who are overweight.

1. Beefsteak

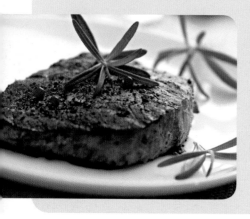

This is one of the most universally available foods that man has. The word beefsteak, which originally comes from America, can refer to many forms or cuts of meat from cattle, minced beef being one of the most common. For the diet, you can find minced beefsteak with a low fat content.

General nutritional characteristics
Beefsteak is very high protein content (20g per 100g); however, the fat content may vary between 5% and 20%. As the amount of fat increases, the protein content decreases. When eaten as part of the Dukan Diet, only steak with between 5% and 10% fat content can be considered. This meat contains 180 calories on average per 100g.

Role in the Dukan Diet
Beefsteak is a great classic and you can ring the changes by selecting different cuts such as skirt of beef, rump steak, flank, top rump, topside and chuck steak. When dieting, minced beef is a great asset as it can be prepared in so many different ways; for example, steak tartare, meatballs, Middle Eastern-style keftas and so on.

How to prepare and eat beefsteak in the Dukan Diet
Beefsteak can be eaten grilled or fried. Flavour it with garlic and parsley, or spice it up by adding a few shallots and a homemade tomato sauce. If preparing minced beefsteak, add some dried herbes de Provence, thyme or rosemary, or make meatballs and add garlic and onions. You can buy minced beefsteak fresh or frozen (but do check the fat content carefully). As with other types of steak, allow it to thaw for several hours in the fridge before cooking it.

Meat loaf
Pain de viande

1 shallot	Salt and black pepper	**Phase 1 PP / Phase 2 PP**
½ bunch of fresh parsley	Tandoori spices	
1 garlic clove	A few cornichons ,	**Preparation time: 15 minutes**
200g (7oz) minced	(small gherkins) to serve	**Cooking time: 45 minutes**
beefsteak (5% fat)		**2 servings**
150g (5½oz) minced		
lean veal		
1 egg		
A little skimmed milk		

Preheat the oven to 180°C/350°F/Gas 4.

Peel the shallot and whizz in a blender, then add the parsley until it is all chopped up and finally the garlic clove.

Add the minced beef and minced veal, then the egg. Blend thoroughly and add a little milk. Season with salt and black pepper and mix in the Tandoori spices.

Turn the mixture out into a medium-sized dish, shape into a loaf and bake in the oven for about 45 minutes.

On the first day eat it warm, then on the following days you can serve it cold with a few cornichons.

2. Bresaola, air-dried/ wind-dried beef

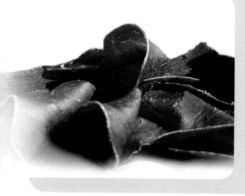

An Italian speciality dating back to the 15th century, when it was common to cure meats by either salting or drying them. Bresaola is dried beef, from which the fat has been removed and the lean meat has been seasoned with salt and spices and dried for between one and three months. It is then sliced as thinly as possible.

General nutritional characteristics

Wind-dried beef is one of the foods with the highest possible protein content (32g per 100g), even higher than the beef it is derived from, since it is dried, dehydrated and the protein content is artificially increased. As it contains so much protein, it will make you feel very full and satisfied.

The Swiss speciality known as viande des Grisons boasts a protein content as high as 40g per 100g; it is available vacuum-packed, as are other types of dried meats. However, it is very important that, when buying dried meats other than bresaola or viande des Grisons, you check they have not been produced with added sugar as this will bump up the calories. Always read the label very carefully.

Role in the Dukan Diet

Full of flavour, bresaola and wind-dried meats in general play an important role in my diet because, in addition to their high protein content, they are delicious and very practical. Easy to carry around with you and easy to use, they should always be stocked in your fridge. If you can find a deli that will slice some bresaola for you as thinly as possible, even better!

How to prepare and eat wind-dried meat in the Dukan Diet

You can eat this meat arranged on a plate with some cornichons (small gherkins), and also with melon in the Consolidation phase. You can enjoy it in a Dukan sandwich or on oat bran galettes too, or alternatively try making it into rolls stuffed with virtually fat-free quark and some fresh herbs of your choice.

Dukan bresaola roll

Roulé de viande des Grisons Dukan

½ cucumber
100g (3½oz) fat-free
   fromage frais
1 garlic clove, crushed
A little lemon juice
Salt and black pepper
100g (3½oz) sliced bresaola

Phase 2 PV

**Preparation time: 5 minutes +
   1 hour chilling
2 servings**

Peel the cucumber and cut into small pieces, removing the central section. Combine with the fromage frais and add the garlic, a few drops of lemon juice, salt and black pepper. Leave this mixture in the fridge for 1 hour to chill and thicken slightly.

Spread the chilled cucumber mixture over the bresaola slices, then roll them up. Use wooden cocktail sticks to keep the rolls in place.

3. Calf's liver

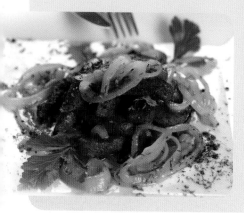

Calf's liver is a very prized piece of offal that holds a place of honour in a butcher's shop. It is also one of the most expensive you can buy. Make sure that you are buying genuine calf's liver and that you are not confusing it with cow's liver.

General nutritional characteristics

Very rich in proteins (24g per 100g), calf's liver contains a lot of vitamins – (B3), B12 and A – as well as iron.

Role in the Dukan Diet

Lean, full of flavour, tender and highly nutitious, calf's liver has the only drawbacks of containing an awful lot of cholesterol and being an organ, described as offal, which some people may find off-putting. You are recommended to eat it once a week, unless you suffer from cholesterol problems or gout.

How to prepare and eat calf's liver in the Dukan Diet

Calf's liver is served in pan-fried slices, but take care to cook it over a very low heat, because if you sear it, it will shrink and harden. Add salt only once it is cooked. You could also try the classic French dish *foie à la vénitienne*, which uses onions and vinegar.

Calf's liver with raspberry vinegar

Foie de veau au vinaigre de framboise

1 small onion, thinly sliced
1 shallot, chopped
2 x 175g (6oz) slices
  calf's liver
Salt and black pepper
2 tablespoons raspberry
  vinegar
2 teaspoons fresh thyme
1 bay leaf

Phase 1 PP / Phase 2 PP

Preparation time: 3 minutes
Cooking time: 12 minutes
2 servings

Gently fry the onion and shallot in a non-stick frying pan. Once they are nicely golden brown, transfer them to a plate and keep to one side.

Now place the calf's liver slices in the frying pan and cook for about 4 minutes on each side. Season with salt and pepper. Transfer to a warm dish and cover to keep hot.

Return the onion mixture to the frying pan and add the raspberry vinegar, thyme and bay leaf. Heat for 2 minutes, stirring continually, then add the liver to warm through in the sauce. Serve straightaway.

4. Fat-reduced bacon

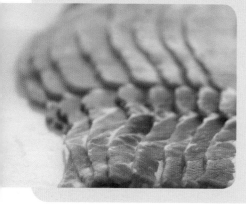

Bacon is one of the most evocative words in Anglo-Saxon gastronomy. Unfortunately, traditional bacon is too fatty to be allowed in the Dukan Diet, which allows only oils from cold-water oily fish. However, it can be very easily substituted with extra-lean pork or turkey bacon.

General nutritional characteristics
A rasher of extra-lean pork bacon weighing 13g contains 21 calories, including 0.8 cal of fat. As for extra-lean turkey bacon, a rasher that weighs 15g – slightly over ½ ounce – contains only 20 calories, including 5g fat.

Role in the Dukan Diet
Bacon symbolizes the spontaneity of a traditional breakfast and brings to mind diet-free times. All you need is a rasher or two of bacon and you can start the day off without feeling any sense of restriction; bacon brightens up your diet with its lovely colour and savoury, smoky taste.

How to prepare and eat fat-reduced bacon in the Dukan Diet
In my diet, smoked, extra-lean bacon teams up beautifully with fried eggs and enlivens salads. For those who have to watch their cholesterol, why not try fried egg whites garnished with whole bacon rashers or small bacon strips.

Dukan hamburger
Hamburger Dukan

2 tablespoons oat bran
1 egg
2 tablespoons fat-free fromage frais
1 teaspoon baking powder
1 onion, chopped
1 minced beef burger (5% fat)
2 slices fat-reduced bacon
Mustard

Sugar-free ketchup or Dukan mayonnaise (see page 222)
1 cornichon, sliced
1 tomato slice
1 red onion, sliced

Phase 2 PV

Preparation time: 10 minutes
Cooking time: 10 minutes, or more depending on preference
1 serving

To make your burger bun, mix together the oat bran, egg, fromage frais and baking powder. Place the dough in a round mould and bake for 4 minutes in a microwave oven. Turn the bun out of the mould and cut in half. If you prefer your bun to be crispier, you can lightly toast it.

In a non-stick frying pan, soften the chopped onion in a little water and then add your beef burger and cook to your preferred doneness. Once it is cooked, lightly fry the low-fat bacon.

Spread a little mustard over one half of the bun then add some sugar-free ketchup or Dukan mayonnaise, according to your taste. Next place the burger and bacon slices on top. Finally, add the cornichon, tomato and red onion, then top with the other bun half and enjoy!

5. Fillet of Beef

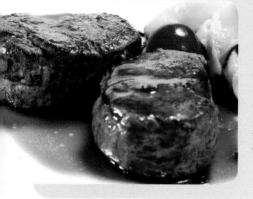

Fillet is the most tender, most sophisticated and most flavoursome cut of beef, which makes it the most sought after and also the most expensive! Fillet can also be cut into Chateaubriand steaks (the heart of the fillet) and tournedos steaks. Depending on the animal and how it was bred, the fillet may also be ideal for roasting.

General nutritional characteristics
Fillet of beef is very high in proteins (20g per 100g). Its fat content may vary between 5% and 15% (generally it is 10%) and it contains 180 calories per 100g.

Role in the Dukan Diet
A meat to keep for special occasions. Different countries all have various ways of cooking it, so there is a wide range of recipes available.

How to prepare and eat fillet of beef in the Dukan Diet
The traditional way to eat fillet of beef is to pan-fry it or roast it whole as a joint. In the Consolidation and Stabilization phases, beef stroganoff or *filet en croûte* make a wonderful treat.

Tiger's tears
Larmes du tigre

2 × 150g (5½oz) fillets of beef
Fresh coriander, finely
  chopped
Thai (garlic) chives, finely
  chopped

For the marinade
3 tablespoons oyster sauce
1 tablespoon soy sauce

1 tablespoon cognac
1 garlic clove, crushed
1 teaspoon mustard seeds,
  crushed

For the sauce
2 tablespoons lime juice
1 teaspoon fish sauce
½ teaspoon liquid sweetener

Phase 1 PP / Phase 2 PP

Preparation time: 5 minutes +
  5 hours marinating
Cooking time: 6 minutes
2 servings

First prepare the marinade by mixing together all the ingredients. Soak the fillets of beef in the marinade for at least 5 hours, covered with clingfilm. Halfway through, turn the meat over.

Make the sauce by combining all the ingredients.

Using a frying pan preferably with a thick cast-iron bottom, cook the meat until it is medium rare, then slice it thinly and pour over the sauce. Sprinkle with the finely chopped coriander and Thai chives, and serve.

6. Game

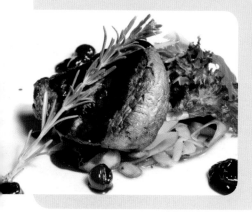

Game covers meat from wild animals and those not raised as domesticated livestock. All types of game have fed on unpolluted foods, so what they have in common is firm, lean flesh packed with good-quality proteins, which makes game a great ally for dieters.

General nutritional characteristics

Nutritionally, ordinary game provides only around 100 calories per 100g, which puts it on a par with low-fat fish – with the one important advantage that its flesh is far more dense and filling.

Role in the Dukan Diet

Obviously game is a food that comes highly recommended in my diet, but there are four minor limitations: its strong taste, price, seasonal availability, and the fact that it is almost compulsory to serve it with some sort of sauce. As regards taste, go for the youngest animal possible; price, find someone who goes hunting!; seasonal availability, use your freezer and frozen products; sauces, try to serve roasts, use sauces made with low-fat fromage frais and go to town with herbs, spices and marinades.

How to prepare and eat game in the Dukan Diet

You will have to roast some cuts from certain young animals, while some game birds such as pheasant and other really tender pieces of meat are especially nice if you marinate them. The most prized game includes large hares, venison and wild boar, which do have to be cooked in a sauce. To enjoy the most important thing – the actual taste and texture of the meat – you can always take it out of the sauce!

Venison stew
Civet de biche

800g (1lb 12oz) stewing
  venison
250ml (9fl oz) red wine
  (tolerated)
250ml (9fl oz) water
4 carrots
2 shallots
3 onions
4 cloves

10 coriander seeds
10 pink peppercorns
2 pinches of ground ginger
½ teaspoon ground allspice
4 bay leaves
1 sprig fresh thyme
1 sprig fresh rosemary
Salt and black pepper

Phase 2 PV

**Preparation time: 10 minutes +
  overnight marinating
Cooking time: 2 hours**
4 servings

Marinate the venison overnight in the wine along with all the other ingredients. The next day, remove the meat and brown it in a cast-iron casserole.

Pour in the marinade juices and leave to simmer, uncovered, for 1 hour, then cover and simmer for a further hour.

Serve on to warmed plates with puréed Romanesco broccoli/cauliflower or celeriac, or perhaps some baked fennel.

7. Kidney

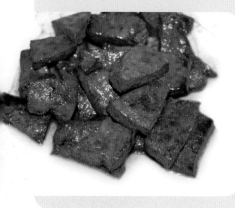

Kidneys are offal, and they can taste very delicate, subtle and delicious.

General nutritional characteristics
Kidneys have a high protein content (17g per 100g) and are very rich in iron and vitamin B12. Unfortunately, as they contain a lot of cholesterol and uric acid, they should not be eaten by anyone at risk from cardiovascular disease, gout, or who suffers from too much uric acid.

Role in the Dukan Diet
The level of tenderness and subtlety of flavour are directly linked to the age of the animal and this is why calf's kidneys are the most sought after. Try to eat kidneys that are as light in colour as possible; if they are almost beige, this indicates that the calf was fed with nothing other than milk. The redder the kidney is in colour, the stronger and less pleasant the taste will be.

How to prepare and eat kidneys in the Dukan Diet
Either grill or pan-fry kidneys with some salt and thyme – use kitchen paper to smear a tiny spoonful of oil over the pan. Try making kebabs with kidneys and serve with sautéed tomatoes and watercress. Kidneys can be expensive.

Tomato kidneys with Dukan bran

Rognons à la tomate et son Dukan

200g (7oz) veal or beef
  kidneys
4 tomatoes peeled, or
  ½ × 400g tin
Salt and black pepper
1 tablespoon wheat bran
1 tablespoon oat bran

Phase 2 PV

Preparation time: 3 minutes
Cooking time: 12–15 minutes
2 servings

Cook the kidneys in a non-stick frying pan until they start to take on some colour. Add the tomatoes, salt, black pepper and, if required, a little water, and cook until this mixture reduces.

Once the kidneys are cooked, pour in a little more water and add the wheat and oat bran to thicken the sauce slightly and bring out the flavour.

8. Pre-cooked ham slices (without any fat or rind)

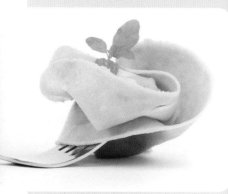

This sort of low-fat ham has revolutionized the snack foods available to consumers in supermarkets. It is full of flavour, reliable and manufactured by major brands that are able to produce it safely.

General nutritional characteristics
As far as nutrition goes, low-fat ham slices have few calories (120 per 100g), and lots of protein (20g per 100g) with 4g fat per 100g. Along with low-fat chicken and turkey slices, it has one of the best statistical profiles of all the Dukan foods.

Role in the Dukan Diet
Sliced ham is extremely useful and very popular because it is so handy. For anyone who does not have a canteen at work nor the time or the money to eat out, it makes a good lunch. Those who eat sliced ham all the time say that, as long as they ring the changes and eat it along with other meats such as turkey and chicken, they do not grow tired of it.

How to prepare and eat pre-cooked ham slices in the Dukan Diet
Well sealed in vacuum packs, sliced ham is easy to carry around and can be eaten anywhere, in the office, in the car, without it smelling or being an inconvenience. More often than not, ham slices are eaten just as they are from the pack at mealtimes, but you can cook with them too. Sliced ham works well in omelettes, especially those made with egg whites only – you just add in some finely chopped ham. Another nice dish is ham wrapped around braised chicory and cooked in the oven with a sauce. Then there is ham soufflé and, of course, it makes a great topping for the Dukan oat bran pizza.

Ham with chicory and Dukan béchamel sauce

Endives au jambon béchamel Dukan

500ml (18fl oz) skimmed milk	A little low-fat Gruyère cheese, grated	**Phase 2 PV**
40g (1½oz) cornflour		
Salt and black pepper		**Preparation time: 10 minutes**
Generous pinch of grated nutmeg		**Cooking time: 20 minutes**
4 chicory heads		**2 servings**
4 slices pre-cooked ham, without any fat or rind		

Preheat the oven to 180°C/350°F/Gas 4.

Meanwhile, make the béchamel sauce. Pour the cold milk into a pan and sprinkle in the cornflour. Stir together with a spatula and place over a gentle heat, stirring until the sauce thickens. Add salt, black pepper and nutmeg.

Pour a little of béchamel sauce into a gratin dish. Wrap each chicory head in a slice of ham and place in the dish. Pour the rest of the sauce over the ham-wrapped chicory.

Sprinkle with the Gruyère cheese and bake in the oven for 15 minutes.

9. Rabbit

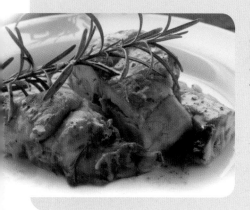

Farmed rabbit is a source of really delicious meat and it is very popular in France. Its one downside, for those who are lazy or do not have much time, is that you have to prepare it.

General nutritional characteristics

Rabbit meat is lean, full of good proteins (22g per 100g of saddle of rabbit). As rabbits feed on alfalfa, their meat is rich in omega 3.

Role in the Dukan Diet

Having to spend some time preparing a rabbit is to my mind a great advantage because by getting involved like this you work at producing a greater variety of flavours. With rabbit, you can also buy different cuts, so there is a wide range of different tastes and textures available. Rabbit meat is also lovely and firm; it requires some chewing but at the same time it is a tasty, tender and enjoyable meat. Finally, most budgets can stretch to rabbit.

How to prepare and eat rabbit in the Dukan Diet

The absolute classic French recipe is rabbit with mustard, a dish that even children adore because the mustard loses its sharp taste once it is cooked. Rabbit can be cooked in the oven, in foil parcels, as kebabs and on the barbecue. Saddle of rabbit is usually most people's favourite cut. Rabbit is also good for making the very leanest terrines. If you are using minced meat in a recipe, you should always consider trying rabbit.

Rabbit with mustard
Lapin à la moutarde

1 good-sized whole rabbit
White wine vinegar
2 tablespoons balsamic
  vinegar
1 onion, diced
Salt and black pepper
Fresh parsley, chopped
3 tablespoons mustard

Phase 1 PP / Phase 2 PP

Preparation time: 15 minutes
**Cooking time: 20 minutes in a
  pressure cooker**
2–3 servings

Chop up the rabbit, clean it and remove any fat. Wash in the white wine vinegar, rinse and then wipe the pieces dry.

Place a large pressure cooker over a high heat and add the balsamic vinegar.

Add the rabbit pieces to brown them, moving them around. After about 5 minutes, add the onion, salt, black pepper and some chopped parsley and cook for a further 5 minutes.

Stir in the mustard and place the lid on the pressure cooker. Once it has reached pressure, cook the rabbit for 15 minutes.

10. Roast beef

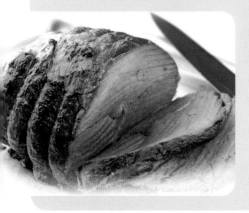

A roast beef joint is a tender cut, boned and sold tied up with string. The best roast beef is taken from the fillet or the sirloin, but it can also come from the flank. For a meat fondue you will need rump steak.

General nutritional characteristics
As far as nutrition goes, the quality of the beef will depend on the cut you have selected but the proteins it contains will always be outstanding, so too its iron and vitamin B12 content.

Role in the Dukan Diet
Roast beef makes a fantastic contribution to my diet as you can enjoy it roasted in its juices one day and then continue eating it sliced cold for the next few days with other cold meats and some mustard. It is tasty, handy for taking in to work, and it makes a nice change from low-fat sliced turkey, chicken and ham.

How to prepare and eat roast beef in the Dukan Diet
Traditionally, a roast beef joint is cooked as a joint in the oven, but there are many casserole recipes too, and there is a whole array of other ingredients that team up well with beef such as Brussels sprouts, carrots, Provençale-style baked tomatoes, onions and low-fat bacon.

Roast beef with garlic sauce
Rosbif au four

4–5 garlic cloves
1 × 1kg (2lb 4oz) roast
  beef joint
Salt and black pepper

Phase 1 PP / Phase 2 PP

Preparation time: 10 minutes
Cooking time: 25–35 minutes
4–6 servings

Preheat the oven to 240°C/475°F/Gas 9.

Peel the garlic cloves and cut one into several very thin slices. Using a pointed knife, prick the joint in several places and insert a slice of garlic into each slit. Place the remaining garlic cloves in the dripping pan.

Place the joint on the top shelf of the oven with the dripping pan below. Allow the joint to sear for 7–8 minutes, then lower the temperature to 220°C/425°F/Gas 7. Cook the joint for 20–25 minutes if you want the meat to be rare inside and add an additional 4 minutes if you prefer your meat cooked à point. Season with salt and freshly ground black pepper once the joint is cooked.

Turn the oven off and allow the meat to rest for 6–8 minutes, leaving the door open. Then take the joint out of the oven and remove the string. Slice the meat on to a warmed serving dish or plate.

Take the dripping pan out of the oven, add a glass of water and scrape up all the cooking juices. Warm through in the pan over a direct heat and add any juices obtained from slicing the meat. Pour the garlic sauce into a gravy boat to serve with the sliced roast beef.

11. Rump steak

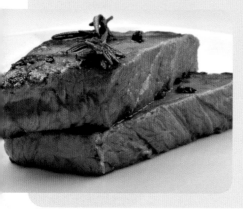

This is one of the most highly recommended meats for my diet. Tender, lean and tasty, it is a great meat for grilling which comes from the ox. It is a lean cut that has short, muscular fibres.

General nutritional characteristics

Rump steak is one of the leanest and best cuts of the animal. It has 4–5g of fat per 100g and is rich in proteins, iron and zinc. It outshines any competition from those 5%-fat steak burgers, which are never as nice.

Role in the Dukan Diet

Rump steak plays an important role in my diet. Often the butcher can separate the rump steak fillet – a cut that is almost as tender as fillet steak and often tastier – from the second part the top rump which is tougher, a little leaner and less tender (it is left to mature for a week before being sold).

How to prepare and eat rump steak in the Dukan Diet

Traditionally, rump steak is sliced and grilled, or it can be cut into cubes and made into kebabs. You can also buy it frozen, but you will need to allow 6–7 hours for the meat to thaw in the fridge.

Rump steak Provençale
Rumsteck à la provençale

2 small aubergines	Fresh parsley, chopped	**Phase 2 PV**
½ red pepper, diced		
3 garlic cloves, thinly sliced		**Preparation time: 30 minutes**
1 onion, finely chopped		**Cooking time: 12–15 minutes**
2 plum tomatoes, chopped		**2 servings**
½ teaspoon mild paprika		
½ teaspoon dried oregano		
Salt and black pepper		
300g (10½oz) rump steak		

Preheat the oven to 200°C/400°F/Gas 6.

Wash and wipe dry the aubergines, without removing the stalks. Slice lengthways into a fan shape. Sprinkle some salt over each slice and put to one side for 20 minutes.

Cover the bottom of a pan with some water and gently cook the red pepper, garlic and onion. Add the plum tomatoes, paprika and oregano and leave to simmer for 5 minutes. Season with salt and black pepper, stir well and put to one side.

Cut the meat into thin strips.

Rinse the aubergine slices and arrange them in an ovenproof dish. Cook 10 minutes in the oven, turning them over carefully several times. Take the dish out of the oven, spread 1 tablespoon of the tomato mixture over each aubergine slice and place a strip of meat on top. Put back in the oven and cook for 20 minutes. Serve immediately, sprinkled with some chopped fresh parsley.

12. Sirloin steak

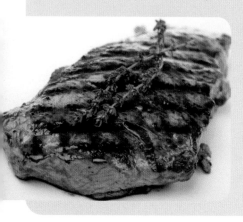

Sirloin is the cut of beef that lies just above the fillet, which is why in French it is called *faux-filet*, or 'false fillet'. It is slightly marbled, with more fat than the fillet, and is a little less tender. This is the meat used for the famous *churrasco* eaten in South America.

General nutritional characteristics

Very rich in proteins (20g per 100g), sirloin steak is also a good source of iron (3mg/100g) and B vitamins.

Role in the Dukan Diet

Sirloin is a really useful food, being such a good source of proteins and iron; a 100g steak, after it has been digested, provides as much iron as 2 kilos of spinach.

How to prepare and eat sirloin steak in the Dukan Diet

Sirloin can be cooked in so many different ways and is mostly roasted or grilled. As with all red meat, take care to grill it as quickly as possible over a high heat or roast it in a very hot oven so that you create an impermeable 'crust' that seals in all the meat juices. Add seasoning only midway through the cooking so that the juices and blood do not disappear. You can also buy frozen slices and joints.

Marinated and grilled sirloin steak

Le faux-filet mariné et grillé

1 garlic clove
1 piece (5cm/2inch) fresh ginger, peeled
300ml (10fl oz) balsamic vinegar
1 small bouquet garni
½ teaspoon ground allspice
1 teaspoon mustard

Pinch of salt
½ teaspoon mustard seeds, crushed
1 × 500g (1lb 2oz) thick sirloin steak
Fresh chervil, finely chopped

Phase 1 PP / Phase 2 PP

Preparation time: 20 minutes + 5 hours marinating
Cooking time: 4 minutes
2 servings

First make the marinade. Crush the garlic and ginger in a shallow dish. Add the balsamic vinegar, bouquet garni, allspice, mustard, salt and crushed mustard seeds.

Cut the sirloin steak in two and place in the marinade. Cover with clingfilm and leave to marinate for 5 hours, turning the slices over halfway through.

When ready to cook, remove the meat from the marinade, drain and wipe with some kitchen paper. Retain half of the marinade and strain it through a sieve. Pour into a pan and simmer over a low heat to reduce slightly.

Heat a non-stick grill pan and cook the sirloin slices for 3–4 minutes on each side. Leave to rest for 5 minutes covered with aluminium foil.

In the meantime, finish off the sauce by warming through the reduced marinade. Adjust the seasoning, then pour over the meat and serve straightaway with some chervil sprinkled on top.

13. Tongue

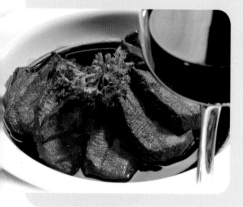

Tongue is commonly available and the only offal we eat tinned. It's impossible to be indifferent about tongue – you either love it or you hate it!

General nutritional characteristics
With a good protein content (17g per 100g), relatively low in fat (10g per 100g), tongue is quite lean. It is the offal with the least cholesterol, but also the least iron.

Role in the Dukan Diet
If you like beef tongue, it allows you to add some variety to your meats and sources of protein. If you are at risk from cardiovascular disease, you should eat it in moderation.

How to prepare and eat tongue in the Dukan Diet
Generally, tongue is served with a piquant (spicy) or tomato sauce, or stewed with vegetables.

Beef tongue with piquant sauce
Langue de boeuf sauce piquante

1 beef tongue
4 tablespoons plus 1 glass
   white wine vinegar
2 low-salt beef stock cubes
1 tablespoon cornflour
1 × 142g tin tomato purée
Dash of harissa
10 cornichons (small
   gherkins), thinly sliced

Phase 1 PP / Phase 2 PP

Preparation time: 15 minutes
Cooking time: 2 hours 40 minutes
2 servings

Rinse the beef tongue in cold water and leave to soak for 15 minutes in fresh cold water to which you have added a glass of white wine vinegar.

Then drain the tongue, place it in a casserole and cover with more fresh cold water. Add the stock cubes, bring to the boil,and simmer for 2½ hours, skimming off any foam at regular intervals.

Once the tongue is cooked, remove it from the stock. Take off the skin; it should come away easily. Cut the tongue into even slices and arrange them in a dish, covering them with a little of the stock so that the meat does not dry out. Keep warm.

Strain the remaining stock through a sieve. Make the sauce by mixing the cornflour with a glass of the strained stock and, once this is thoroughly combined, add a second glass followed by three more glasses of stock. Warm over a medium heat until the sauce starts to thicken, whisking all the time. Then add the tomato purée, the 4 tablespoons of vinegar, a dash of harissa and the thinly sliced cornichons.

14. Veal chop

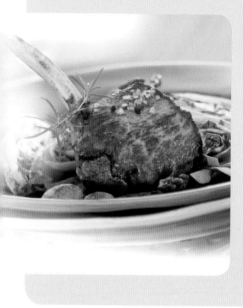

This is a highly prized piece of meat. It is much less fatty than rib of beef (which is not allowed in the diet) and therefore less flavoursome. Remember that the chop will vary depending on where it has been taken from. The first chop that gets cut is the fleshiest, but is a bit fatty at the sides. The second chop is even fattier, but its eye is not quite as good. The exposed chop is not as wide, has more fibrous membranes and is firmer. The fillet chop has its T-shaped bone and matching piece of fillet. This is the biggest chop and the one best suited to those with a hearty appetite. Without the fillet, this is the classic veal chop.

General nutritional characteristics

Veal chops contain a lot of protein (24g per 100g) and are a good source of zinc, iron, phosphorus and vitamins B12 and PP. Chops are the cut of veal with the most fat (15.4g per 100g).

Role in the Dukan Diet

Provided you carefully remove the layer of fat on the side away from the bone, which does take a little time, this is a lean meat and very useful in the diet.

How to prepare and eat veal chops in the Dukan Diet

Remember to take your veal chop out of the fridge 30 minutes before you want to use it, because cold meat does not cook so well. Veal chops can be cooked in the oven in foil parcels or fried in a non-stick pan with the juice of half a lemon, some sliced onions, courgettes (either diced or cut into strips), a few basil leaves and some chives.

Victoria's veal chops
Côtes de veau victoriennes

1 x 400g tin chopped tomatoes
150g (5½oz) carrots, grated
150g (5½oz) celery, chopped
1 teaspoon chopped fresh
 basil
Salt and black pepper
2 veal chops

Phase 2 PV

Preparation time: 15 minutes
Cooking time: 40–50 minutes
2 servings

Preheat the oven to 180°C/350°F/Gas 4.

Pour the tinned tomatoes into a bowl. Add the carrots, celery, basil, salt and black pepper and mix together. Spoon half into the bottom of a small ovenproof dish, place the veal chops on top, then finish off with the remaining tomato mixture.

Cook in the oven for 40–50 minutes.

15. Veal escalope

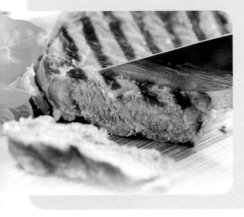

An extremely lean yet very tender piece of meat, veal escalope needs to be cooked in a way that brings out the flavour so that it does not taste insipid. It will lose its tenderness if cooked over too high a heat.

General nutritional characteristics

Very lean indeed (2.5g fat per 100g) and extremely rich in proteins (31g per 100g), veal escalope is also packed with vitamin B12.

Role in the Dukan Diet

Veal escalope, on a par with turkey escalope, allows you to ring the changes as well as providing some top-quality proteins. You can choose escalopes that come from three different cuts: you will get the most tender escalope from very fine-grained meat; then there is the cushion of veal which is just as tender (escalopes taken from here are smaller); and leg of veal provides a larger escalope with a coarser grain which is less tender.

How to prepare and eat veal escalope in the Dukan Diet

A simple way to prepare an escalope is to cook it over a gentle heat and add a sauce made from garlic and chopped onions cooked in tomato passata with some spices and seasoning. You then finish it off in the oven. Veal escalopes can also be prepared with a few herbs and then pan-fried, or breaded and gently fried – you can coat them with a mixture made from an egg yolk, some oat bran and a little very low-fat cream.

Dukan veal Milanese
Escalope de veau milanaise Dukan

2 eggs
Salt and black pepper
2 tablespoons oat bran
2 very thin slices veal escalope
   (150g/5oz each)
1 lemon
Fresh parsley, chopped

Phase 1 PP / Phase 2 PP

Preparation time: 5 minutes
Cooking time: 6 minutes
2 servings

Beat the eggs in a shallow dish and season with salt and black pepper.
Pour the oat bran on to a plate. First dip the escalopes into the egg
mixture, then place them in the bran, making sure both sides are covered.

Very quickly dip the escalopes in the egg mixture once more and then
again in the oat bran so that they are thickly coated.

Add three drops of oil to a frying pan, then wipe away with some kitchen
paper and heat the pan. Place the escalopes in the pan and cook for
3 minutes on each side.

Serve with a squeeze of lemon juice, some chopped parsley and a few
lemon slices.

16. Chicken

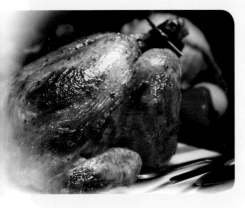

In our modern times, chicken has become a major animal foodstuff since it is now farmed on such a large scale. Most of the chickens we eat, especially if on a tight budget, are young intensively reared birds from the supermarket. Chicken provides nutritionally correct food that is filling and cheap.

General nutritional characteristics
As far as nutrition is concerned, chicken is a relatively lean food (6g fat per 100g; by removing the skin you lose a further 1.5g). Low in calories, it provides up to 140 per 100g (with the skin removed).

Role in the Dukan Diet
In my diet, chicken is a master food, being highly adaptable and easy to use. If you can afford it, buy a free-range or organic whole chicken; you will enjoy far better-quality meat and flavour. Otherwise, you can take your pick: appetizing chicken breasts, drumsticks, wings without the skin, fresh or frozen birds or a ready-cooked chicken – the quality of these is generally quite acceptable.

How to prepare and eat chicken in the Dukan Diet
Chicken is cooked in a whole variety of different ways; each country and culture has its own methods. In France, as in the UK, we like whole roast chicken with its skin and juices. Everyone tends to add their own favourite seasonings, spices and stuffing. Remember that lemons go fantastically well with chicken.

Chicken strips in cider vinegar
Aiguillettes de poulet au vinaigre de cidre

500g (1lb 2oz) chicken, cut
into strips
Salt and black pepper
½ teaspoon ground ginger
Chopped fresh parsley and
garlic mixture (*persillade*)
100ml (3½fl oz) cider vinegar

Phase 1 PP / Phase 2 PP

Preparation time: 5 minutes
Cooking time: 20 minutes
2 servings

In a non-stick frying pan, sear and gently fry the chicken strips.
As soon as they turn golden brown, season with salt and pepper.
Sprinkle over the ground ginger and some *persillade*, then add the
cider vinegar and stir to deglaze the pan (loosen all the browned meat
juices stuck to the bottom).

Leave to cook for at least 5 minutes in the juices, turning the strips over
occasionally. Serve on warmed plates with a little extra *persillade* on top.

17. Chicken liver

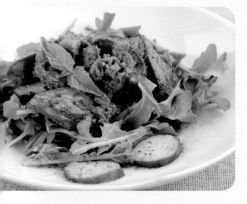

A food that offers great nutritional quality, chicken liver is greatly enjoyed for its unusual flavour and is available at a price that everyone can afford.

General nutritional characteristics
Chicken liver is lean (5g fat per 100g), high in protein (20g per 100g) and really low in calories. It is also a concentrated source of vitamin A and the B vitamins, and is packed with iron, so has the power to stimulate and energize, which when you are dieting is very welcome indeed.

Role in the Dukan Diet
Chicken liver is a master food in my diet as it is one of the five most filling and satisfying foods there are. As it is lean, and stuffed with proteins and a rare supply of vitamins, it is the ideal foodstuff for those lucky enough to enjoy the taste and who do not suffer from high cholesterol.

How to prepare and eat chicken liver in the Dukan Diet
There are many different ways to prepare chicken livers but for the dieter the most enjoyable is to pan-fry them, then to finish off by deglazing with cider or balsamic vinegar. Do not worry about the amount of vinegar – you can never use too much! Chicken livers also work really well in mixed salads and team up very successfully with frisée lettuce. Or you can try a wonderful chicken liver terrine with glazed onions and a few bay leaves to enhance the flavour.

Chicken livers with mixed dried herbs

Foie de volaille aux herbes de Provence

1 tin chicken livers (approx
  250g/9oz)
Salt and black pepper
1 tablespoon balsamic vinegar
1 × 230g tin chopped tomatoes
Herbes de Provence

Phase 2 PV

**Preparation time: 5 minutes
Cooking time: 15 minutes
2 servings**

Gently fry the chicken livers in a non-stick frying pan over a medium heat until they turn golden brown. Season with salt and black pepper. Deglaze the livers with the balsamic vinegar.

Add the chopped tomatoes, season with the herbes de Provence and leave to simmer for 15 minutes.

18. Guinea fowl

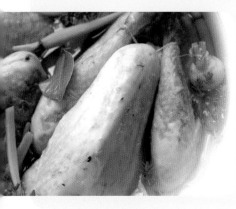

For the French, guinea fowl is what poultry is all about and we are the world's leading producer. Unlike chicken, guinea fowl cannot cope with intensive farming. So a guinea fowl is a bird that has always been properly farmed, then slaughtered when 80 days old.

General nutritional characteristics
Guinea fowl is one of the leanest birds there is (5g fat per 100g); its fats are high-quality (unsaturated), it has the highest protein content and has only 155 calories per 100g.

Role in the Dukan Diet
However, in my diet it is a second-rank food that we do not think of cooking all that often as it requires careful preparation beforehand. So if you come home from work starving and desperate to eat straightaway, guinea fowl does not quite fit the bill.

How to prepare and eat guinea fowl in the Dukan Diet
You should cook guinea fowl in a casserole as its meat is too dry to be roasted in the oven. Cook it with as many vegetables as possible and preferably those with a high water content so that the juices flow around the meat and help keep it nice and moist.

Guinea fowl with cabbage
Pintade au chou

1 × 1.25–1.5kg (2lb 12oz–3lb
   5oz) guinea fowl
4 cloves
1 onion, quartered
6 carrots, thinly sliced
300g (10½oz) chicken, cut into
   thin strips
200g (7oz) button mushrooms
1 × 400g tin chopped tomatoes

1 bouquet garni
1 large cabbage, blanched
1 low-salt chicken stock cube
Salt and black pepper

Phase 2 PV

Preparation time: 30 minutes
**Cooking time: 30 minutes in
   a pressure cooker**
6 servings

Gently fry the guinea fowl in a pressure cooker. It needs to be
golden brown.

Stick a clove in each onion quarter and add to the guinea fowl with
the carrots, chicken strips, mushrooms, chopped tomatoes and bouquet
garni. Add the blanched cabbage and cover with water. Crumble in the
stock cube, stir gently, then season with salt and black pepper.

Put the lid on the pressure cooker and, once the steam has reached
pressure, cook for a further 30 minutes.

19. Ostrich

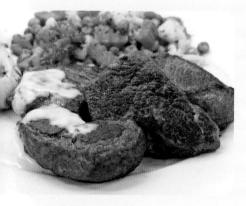

An exotic, unusual meat with a festive touch that will be of interest to anyone who likes something a bit out of the ordinary. What is more, this red, coarse-grained meat is healthy, full of flavour, very tender and has a very high nutritional value.

General nutritional characteristics
When it comes to nutrition, this unusual meat contains fewer calories, less cholesterol and less fat than other meats. Among my 100 foods it has absolute *carte blanche*.

Role in the Dukan Diet
I certainly allow ostrich meat and go as far as heartily recommending it, since it is lean and extremely high in proteins. The only drawback is its price, and the fact that it may not be easily available in all supermarkets.

How to prepare and eat ostrich in the Dukan Diet
You will impress your guests if you try cooking ostrich with a little fat-reduced butter and a teaspoon of port. If you like it tender and on the rare side, the traditional way to cook ostrich is to pan-fry it. Otherwise, you can try it grilled or stewed.

Ostrich carpaccio with basil

Carpaccio d'autruche au basilic

500g (1lb 2oz) ostrich fillets
1 small bunch fresh basil
4 tablespoons olive oil
1 teaspoon olive flavouring
  (www.dukandietshop.co.uk)
Salt and black pepper
A few lettuce leaves, to garnish

Phase 1 PP / Phase 2 PP

Preparation time: 20 minutes
4 servings

Cut the ostrich meat into extremely thin slices.

Wash and finely chop the basil leaves. Make sure they are thoroughly dry. Keep to one side any tiny leaves to use as a garnish. Put the chopped basil, olive oil and flavouring in a blender along with some salt and black pepper and whizz them together so that you get a green sauce that is quite thick and smooth.

Arrange the meat slices on four plates, making sure that the bottom of each plate is covered. Use a small brush to spread a thin layer of the basil sauce over the meat. Give a few twists of black pepper and, in the centre of each plate, arrange some lettuce leaves with the reserved basil leaves.

20. Pigeon

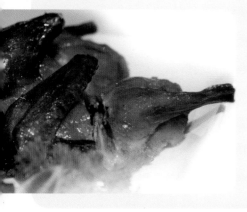

Pigeon is a small bird with delicate meat and is very much appreciated by gourmets. It is unusual, lean, and low in calories and yet you still feel as if you are eating something special, which may also explain why it is expensive.

General nutritional characteristics
Pigeon is one of the best meats for protein (37g per 100g) and it is extremely lean (3g fat per 100g) – you would think that it had been specially created for my diet!

Role in the Dukan Diet
Pigeon is a food that gives my diet a festive and convivial feel; it stops you from thinking that you are dieting. Moreover, it contains an awful lot of protein, which will make you feel full; plus it will take you some time to get all the meat off the bones. Pigeons escape the miseries of intensive industrial rearing and you can tell this from the quality of the meat. Always select a young corn-fed pigeon weighing 400–500g (14oz–1lb 2oz). Finally, wood pigeon or wild pigeon is very sought-after and makes a real celebration.

How to prepare and eat pigeon in the Dukan Diet
As with all small birds, the best way to cook pigeon is in a casserole. Its meat is tender, so it does not need to be cooked for very long. Preserved lemons or chanterelle mushrooms work really well with pigeon, or why not try it stuffed (with veal or beef, mushrooms, shallots, salt and pepper)?

Spicy pigeon
Pigeon aux épices

2 pigeons
Salt and black pepper

For the marinade
2 shallots, chopped
1 garlic clove, chopped
2 cloves
2 pinches of ground cinnamon
2 tablespoons liquid sweetener

1 tablespoon soy sauce
1 tablespoon mustard seeds, crushed

Phase 1 PP / Phase 2 PP

Preparation time: 25 minutes + 2 hours marinating
Cooking time: 30 minutes
2 servings

Ask your butcher to gut the pigeons and keep the livers for you.

In a bowl, combine all the ingredients for the marinade. Place the pigeons in the marinade and leave for 2 hours, making sure you turn them regularly. Then remove the pigeons and keep the marinade.

Preheat the oven to 180°C/350°F/Gas 4.

Season the pigeon livers with salt and black pepper. Gently fry them on both sides in a non-stick frying pan over a medium heat. Chop them up and add half of the marinade. Mix together and use to stuff the pigeons. Truss the birds and cook them in a cast-iron casserole in the oven for about 30 minutes, depending on how big they are, and make sure that you turn them round halfway through.

When they are ready, remove the pigeons from the oven and place them on a warmed serving dish. Put the casserole over a high heat and use the rest of the marinade to deglaze. Pour the sauce into a gravy boat and serve with the birds.

21. Poussin

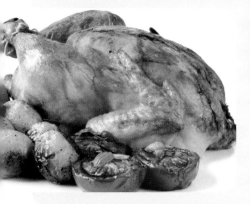

A poussin is a special breed of poultry altogether. Reared to an age of just 32–38 days, on average a poussin weighs around 450g, or 1lb. They can cost about £6–7 a kilo.

General nutritional characteristics
Nutritionally, a poussin is very close to a chicken; it contains a little more protein (21g per 100g), fewer calories (147 per 100g), with a similar fat content (7g with the skin or 6g without).

Role in the Dukan Diet
In my diet, a poussin is a very handy bird for anyone who lives on their own or for couples with a small appetite. A poussin can be cooked quickly, either roasted in the oven or cut in two and grilled or pan-fried.

How to prepare and eat poussin in the Dukan Diet
There are all sorts of ways to cook a poussin. It tastes great spit-roasted, roasted in the oven, grilled or casseroled. The results will vary depending on the bird's quality. If you can afford to spend a little bit more, buy a free-range bird as it will be so much tastier.

Poussins with preserved lemons
Coquelets aux citrons confits

2 poussins
5 sprigs fresh thyme, leaves
  removed
6 preserved lemons, sliced
500ml (18fl oz) chicken stock
2 medium onions, finely
  chopped
2 garlic cloves, chopped
Salt and black pepper

Phase 1 PP / Phase 2 PP

Preparation time: 20 minutes
Cooking time: 40 minutes
2 servings

Preheat the oven to 180°C/350°F/Gas 4.

Place the poussins in an ovenproof dish and sprinkle over the thyme leaves. Cover the birds with the preserved lemon slices and bake in the oven for 20 minutes. After 10 minutes, baste the birds with the chicken stock.

Take the poussins out of the oven and scatter the onions and garlic around them. Season with salt and black pepper, then return the birds to the oven for a further 20 minutes, keeping an eye on them until they are ready.

22. Pre-cooked chicken and turkey slices

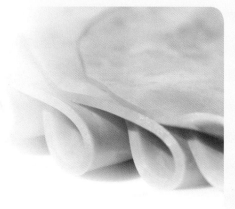

As with pre-cooked ham slices (without any fat or rind), the availability of low-fat sliced poultry has revolutionized what supermarkets can offer the consumer. This cooked meat is tasty, reliable and produced by major brands that have the means to ensure their production is safe. Properly packaged in airtight re-sealable packs, these sliced meats can be taken anywhere and eaten everywhere – in the office, in your car – without annoying others with their smell.

General nutritional characteristics

Nutritionally, this sort of sliced meat contains very few calories (110 per 100g) but lots of protein (22g per 100g), with 2–3g fat per 100g, which means that, along with pre-cooked ham slices without fat and rind, pre-cooked chicken and turkey slices have the best statistics among the Dukan foods.

Role in the Dukan Diet

Since they are so handy at lunchtime, they are extremely practical and widely used. They do not cost too much and if you have neither the time nor the money to eat out every day, or if there is no canteen at work, they make an excellent snack. So that you do not grow tired of eating this sort of sliced meat, try to alternate with other types of cooked meats and try out different varieties (roasted meat, grilled meat, etc.), and include them in cooked recipes too.

How to prepare and eat pre-cooked chicken and turkey slices in the Dukan Diet

This sliced meat is generally eaten just as it comes, straight from the pack. However, you can also use the slices in omelettes or baked in the oven with braised chicory; or you can add them to Dukan sandwiches and eat them with an oat bran galette.

Sliced turkey and chicken rolls
Roulés de jambon de dinde et de poulet

Chopped garlic and fresh
  herbs
100g (3½oz) virtually fat-free
  quark
2 slices pre-cooked turkey
2 slices pre-cooked chicken
Chopped fresh parsley, to
  garnish

Phase 1 PP / Phase 2 PP

Preparation time: 5 minutes
2 servings

Mix the chopped garlic and fresh herbs into the quark.

Lay the pre-cooked turkey and chicken slices flat, then spread the quark
mixture over the slices and roll them up. Cut each roll into six sections
and arrange on a plate.

Scatter over some chopped parsley when ready to serve.

23. Quail

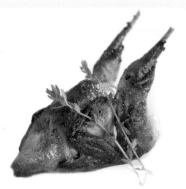

A bird that most people are not very familiar with, quail deserves wider recognition – especially farm-reared quail. Full of protein, with little fat and an average number of calories, this is a bird that suits festive occasions, which was how it was eaten when it used to be a game bird. Now, at last, it is affordable for everyone.

General nutritional characteristics

Nutritionally, a quail is like any other bird and you must remove the skin. A cooked quail contains about 70 calories – about the same amount as you would find in a tub of fat-free yoghurt – along with 4g fat per quail but with 12g of proteins too!

Role in the Dukan Diet

I recommend eating quail in my diet because, if cooked properly, it is full of flavour, delicate and has a good texture; and, above all, it belongs to my 'slow foods' category along with artichokes, crabs, winkles and mussels – foods that all take a long time to eat, that make you feel full, and are therefore particularly good for slowing down any quick eaters.

How to prepare and eat quail in the Dukan Diet

Quail is best cooked in a casserole or roasted in the oven, stuffed with virtually fat-free quark, herbs and seasonings, a teaspoon of oat bran and small pieces of preserved lemon. Try cooking a couple of quails for yourself this way; they will fill you up and leave you satisfied for quite some time.

Quail stuffed with cottage cheese and celeriac purée

Cailles farcies à la faisselle et à la purée de céleri

2 quails
100g (3½oz) fat-free cottage
  cheese
200g (7oz) puréed celeriac
1 bunch of fresh chives,
  chopped
2 pinches of ground cumin
Salt and black pepper

Phase 2 PV

Preparation time: 10 minutes
Cooking time: 15 minutes
2 servings

Preheat the oven to 150°C/300°F/Gas 2.

Debone the quails by the backbone, leaving both sides well attached. Or buy ready-boned birds.

Mix together the cottage cheese, celeriac, chives, cumin, salt and black pepper. Stuff the quails with this mixture, close them up and put them in individual ramekin dishes with the fold underneath. Roast in the oven for 15 minutes.

Serve the quails piping hot with the celeriac stuffing.

24. Turkey

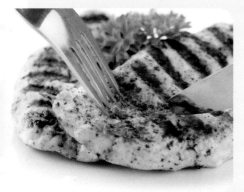

Nowadays turkey is available cheaply everywhere, but for a long time it was a highly prized bird killed only for the Christmas festivities. There is so much more choice, with cheap, large-scale farmed turkeys cut up into crowns, fillets, joints, breasts or pieces for stewing – and you can even buy smaller, farm-raised turkeys for Christmas Day.

General nutritional characteristics
As far as nutrition goes, turkey is the poultry that contains the fewest calories (109 per 100g); it is very lean and very high in protein. It is difficult to make a better choice, as turkey also contains many B vitamins, iron and magnesium, which means that it is energy-giving and calming at the same time.

Role in the Dukan Diet
Turkey plays an important part in my diet as it is the leanest poultry and the leanest of all meats. What is more, it is easy and handy to use. Turkey does not have a lot of flavour, but it does lend itself to all sorts of uses, recipes and cooking methods. To my mind, what tastes best is a nice drumstick roasted in the oven, studded with lots of garlic just like a joint of lamb; you can keep slicing it and eat it over several days. With turkey, you can also produce a very special festive meal and invite others to join you – and all for a really reasonable price.

How to prepare and eat turkey in the Dukan Diet
Turkey breasts are extremely simple to cook with. You can cook them with some Meaux mustard or on a bed of onions, or why not try stuffed turkey (use equal quantities of minced veal, minced beef, pre-cooked ham and sliced mushrooms plus herbs and seasoning to make the stuffing).

Indian-style turkey breasts
Blanc de dinde à l'indienne

2 tablespoons curry powder
200g (7oz) turkey breast meat
Salt and black pepper

Phase 1 PP / Phase 2 PP

Preparation time: 5 minutes
Cooking time: 15 minutes
2 servings

Mix the curry powder with 50ml (2fl oz) water.

Cut the turkey breasts into small pieces and fry them gently in a non-stick frying pan. As soon as they turn golden brown, season with salt and black pepper and add the curry powder mixture. Continue cooking the turkey until all the water has evaporated and serve piping hot.

25. Bass

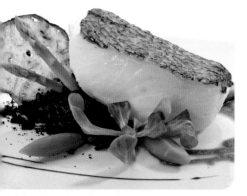

For many, bass is the king of fish because of its fine, sophisticated, white, pearly flesh. It is also relatively lean, making it highly prized but unfortunately very expensive too.

General nutritional characteristics
Bass is lean (1.8g fat per 100g), rich in top-quality proteins (18.5g per 100g) and low in calories (90 per 100g).

Role in the Dukan Diet
In my diet, bass should be regarded as a luxury food, and eating it as an act and a moment of faith which adds a little sparkle to your diet. So keep it for a special family meal or a celebration with friends. For people who eat out on business accounts and do not have to watch their expenses, feel free to order bass or turbot whenever you can!

How to prepare and eat sea bass in the Dukan Diet
Bass flesh is very delicate with a slight seafood taste, so cook it as simply as possible to avoiding spoiling its subtle flavour. Ideally, you would bake it in the oven, whole with fennel seeds and dill – the hint of aniseed combines perfectly with the iodine flavours of the bass. If you have a really big fish, it can also be cooked inside a salt crust (made of flour, salt and water). Use your frying pan only for fillets.

Sea bass with fennel and Pacific sauce

Bar au fenouil et au Pacific

2 × 400g (14oz) sea bass
2 tablespoons Pacific sauce
Salt and black pepper
4 fennel bulbs
Juice of 1 lemon
1 teaspoon ground fennel seed
  or aniseed

Phase 2 PV

Preparation time: 20 minutes
Cooking time: 30 minutes
4 servings

Preheat the oven to 200°C/400°F/Gas 6.

Without descaling the fish, gut them and make 2–3 incisions on each side. Using a small brush, spread 1 tablespoon of the Pacific sauce inside the fish. Season with salt and black pepper. Wash and finely chop the fennel bulbs – keep the fennel leaves to one side. Take one half of the chopped fennel and pour over the lemon juice. Place this fennel inside the fish.

Arrange the bass in a large ovenproof dish. Pour over the remaining tablespoon of Pacific sauce and half a glass of water. Sprinkle with the ground fennel seed or aniseed. Place the remaining chopped fennel around the fish.

Bake in oven for 30 minutes, checking that the fish is not overcooked and basting occasionally with the juices. When ready to serve, garnish with the fennel leaves.

26. Cod

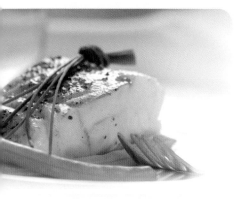

Cod is popular everywhere – it is the epitome of lean, white fish that tastes great and is easy to find. We appreciate its subtle flavour, but even more so its wonderful texture. Cod flesh gives way as soon as you press a fork on it.

General nutritional characteristics

Cod is one of the leanest fish (0.7g fat per 100g), the least calorific (75 calories per 100g) and also the easiest to digest as it contains few connective fibres, which take ages to break down. And yet cod provides as much protein as beef, with a high B vitamin and iodine content too.

Role in the Dukan Diet

Cod, along with sole, is the most popular fish in France; it is the only white fish to have put up a fight and resisted salmon taking over the market. With cod available, following my diet is so much easier. Its price is its only downside, as cod steaks are no longer affordable for everyone.

How to prepare and eat cod in the Dukan Diet

With such delicate flesh, cod tastes fabulous when just cooked briefly in a frying pan on a bed of browned onions. It is also good for making kebabs on the barbecue. Avoid using white wine when cooking cod as this will overpower the subtle flavour of the fish. Those of you with a taste for the exotic, could try salted cod, which is much firmer because of the salt. Soak it for 48 hours in cold water. Then cook it on a griddle, pan-fry or bake it in the oven with tomatoes and peppers. It can also be flaked to make a *brandade*, a creamed salt cod dish. Cod roe can be fried, but people often forget about it, so it ends up in taramasalata. Always try to remember to ask for the fresh roe whenever you visit the fishmonger.

Cod terrine with smoked salmon and scallops

Terrine de cabillaud au saumon fumé et noix de Saint-Jacques

500g (1lb 2oz) fresh cod
Handful of fresh chives
½ small onion
1 egg
150ml (5fl oz) low-fat crème fraîche
½ teaspoon fennel seeds
Black pepper
3 scallops

2 large slices smoked salmon
1 fennel bulb

Phase 2 PV

Preparation time: 15 minutes
Cooking time: 30 minutes
3–4 servings

Preheat the oven to 160°C/325°F/Gas 3 and line a loaf tin with greaseproof paper, leaving a generous overlap along the long sides.

Finely blend the cod in a food processor with the chives and onion, then pour this mixture into a large bowl. Add the egg, crème fraîche and fennel seeds and stir to combine all the ingredients. Season with black pepper.

Dice the scallops. Put aside enough of the cod mixture to cover the bottom of the loaf tin and add the chopped scallops to the remaining mixture.

Spread some of the scallop-free mixture over the bottom of the tin, leaving enough for the top.

Next lay out the smoked salmon slices and spread some of the scallop mixture on top. Roll up the salmon slices and place them on top of the cod mixture in the tin. Cover the top and sides with the remaining cod mixture.

Fold over both sides of the greaseproof paper and bake in the oven for 30 minutes. Once the terrine is cooked, leave to cool and serve cold.

27. Seafood sticks

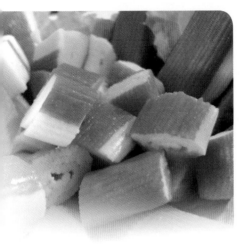

With globalization, this foodstuff is now widely available and can help us tackle weight problems. Seafood sticks originate in Japan, where they are produced out in the fishing grounds on the open seas; the *surimi* base (Japanese for chopped fish) is made from the white meat of extra-lean fish. The Japanese also use it to make imitation shellfish. In France and Europe, it is combined with a binding agent, with starch, some seafood flavouring and egg white. This mixture is then cooked, reduced to strands and lastly shaped into sticks or flakes.

General nutritional characteristics
Nutritionally, this is a high-quality food, clean and safe, despite being the target of unfounded rumours like other foods that people are unsure of. To my mind, and for anyone trying to lose weight, seafood sticks are a top food, with 113 calories per 100g and 4.5g fat per 100g.

Role in the Dukan Diet
In my diet, seafood sticks are a master stroke, as they offer just about every advantage. Easy to carry around, odourless, ready to eat, cheap; their taste is straightforward but easy to get used to; they are filling and satisfying, lean and simple to use in many different ways. Experience has shown that they are among the 45 most used foods, especially for anyone who has to eat lunch in a hurry. They are so useful and make dieting so much less troublesome that the fact they contain 6% slow carbohydrates does not worry me any more than the lactose content in dairy products does.

How to prepare and eat seafood sticks in the Dukan Diet
More often than not, these sticks are eaten on their own or crumbled into salads. With a little imagination, they can be included in all sorts of recipes such as seafood stick appetizers using virtually fat-free quark; leek and seafood stick terrine; tuna and seafood stick loaf, and so on.

Seafood stick gratin
Gratin au surimi

360g (12½oz) seafood sticks,
  grated
2 eggs
115g (4oz) virtually fat-free
  quark
4 tablespoons fat-free fromage
  frais
Salt and black pepper
2 teaspoons agar-agar

Phase 1 PP / Phase 2 PP

Preparation time: 8 minutes
Cooking time: 20 minutes
2 servings

Preheat the oven to 230°C/450°F/Gas 8.

Put the grated seafood sticks into a large bowl and break the eggs over them. Add the quark and fromage frais. Season with salt and black pepper. Stir in the agar-agar and combine all the ingredients thoroughly until the mixture is smooth.

Pour the mixture into a small square or oval ovenproof dish and bake in the oven for 20 minutes until the gratin has risen slightly and turned golden brown.

28. Dab/lemon sole

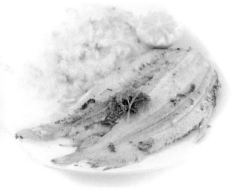

An ultra-lean and low-calorie fish, whose flesh is subtle and delicate but does not require much chewing. It has three main advantages: it is affordable; it is filling because it contains a lot of excellent quality proteins; and it has a strong iodine flavour, which appeals to those who like this taste and is good for anyone who has a lazy thyroid.

General nutritional characteristics
Dab or lemon sole is a lean fish (1g fat per 100g), rich in proteins (18g per 100g), low in calories (73 per 100g) and rich in iodine.

Role in the Dukan Diet
In my diet, dab or lemon sole is recommended only to the converted. People who simply do not like it would never think of eating it or feel motivated to do so. I quite understand this; there are so many fish to choose from and what keeps any diet going is that you are able to get as much pleasure as possible using the foods you are allowed.

How to prepare and eat dab or lemon sole in the Dukan Diet
A dab or lemon sole usually comes as a portion size and is pan-fried following the ritual 'three drops of oil plus kitchen paper'. Cook it for only a brief time over an intense heat so that you maintain as much firmness on the inside as possible while the surface is crispy, seared by the heat from the frying pan.

Lemon sole fillets stuffed with scallops

Filets de limande farcis aux coquilles Saint-Jacques

4 dab or lemon sole fillets
16 scallops
Juice of 3 lemons
Salt and black pepper
1 teaspoon cornflour
2 tablespoons 3% fat cream
A few fresh chives, chopped

Phase 1 PP / Phase 2 PP

Preparation time: 10 minutes
Cooking time: 20 minutes
4 servings

Preheat the oven to 200°C/400°F/Gas 6.

Cut each fillet in two lengthways. Place one scallop on top of each piece and roll it up. Use wooden cocktail sticks to keep the rolls in place and arrange in an ovenproof dish. Place the remaining scallops around the rolled-up fish. Pour over the juice from 1 lemon and season lightly with salt and black pepper. Bake in the oven for 20 minutes.

Meanwhile, warm the juice from the remaining lemons in a pan over a gentle heat. Dissolve the cornflour in 2 tablespoons of water. Once the lemon juice starts to simmer, stir in the cream and, using a whisk, combine thoroughly. Leave on a gentle heat for a few minutes, stirring all the time, then add the dissolved cornflour and stir well as the sauce will start to thicken. Add a little salt and black pepper.

Serve the fish on warmed plates, pour over the sauce and sprinkle with the chives.

29. Dover sole

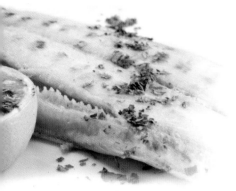

As far as many fish lovers are concerned, Dover sole is the king of fish, with its delicate, white, fine flesh. In my opinion, Dover sole is the fish that people who dislike fish find easiest to try. The same goes for children who learn to enjoy the firm, mild-flavoured flesh, with the added bonus of no bones. This taste then stays with them for life.

General nutritional characteristics

Dover sole is probably about as lean a fish as you can get (0.5g fat per 100g), as high in proteins as the best protein fish and very low in calories (70 per 100g).

Role in the Dukan Diet

Dover sole has an important place in my diet. It is perfect for business lunches and dinners, as it is one of the few fish that chefs are quite happy to grill simply. It is quite expensive, so counts as a luxury fish, and the person eating it can derive some extra symbolic pleasure. Lastly, Dover sole is a fish that can be recommended to people who dislike touching or preparing fish, as they can eat it without feeling anxious about the preparation.

How to prepare and eat Dover sole in the Dukan Diet

Dover sole should be cooked as simply as possible as any extra ingredients could impair its delicate flavour, its most important asset. So either grill it or pan-fry it with some lemon juice. To enhance its subtle flavour even further, try serving it with crayfish and a bisque.

Parcels of Dover sole fillets and prawns

Papillotes de filets de sole et crevettes grises

8 tablespoons fat-free fromage frais
2 tablespoons 3% fat crème fraîche
Salt and black pepper
8 fresh chives, finely chopped
8 Dover sole fillets
2 lemons, thinly sliced
115g (4oz) raw prawns

2 sprigs fresh flat-leaf parsley, leaves removed

Phase 1 PP / Phase 2 PP

Preparation time: 20 minutes
Cooking time: 20 minutes
4 servings

Preheat the oven to 180°C/350°F/Gas 4.

Pour the fromage frais and the crème fraîche into a saucepan. Season with salt and black pepper. Add the chives and warm over a very low heat without allowing the sauce to boil.

Cut out four large squares of greaseproof paper. Roll up the Dover sole fillets and hold in place with wooden cocktail sticks. Place a slice of lemon in the centre of each fillet roll and then place two rolled fillets on each greaseproof paper square. Pour the chive sauce over the rolled-up fillets, then divide the shrimps and parsley leaves between the four parcels.

Seal the parcels, place them on a baking tray in the oven and bake for 18–20 minutes. Serve immediately, piping hot.

30. Grey mullet

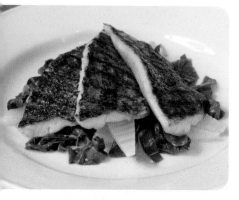

Steel grey and streamlined like a plane, grey mullet is a very fine fish. It is muscular, quick and lively, with firm, white and beautiful flesh. Grey mullet can be prepared in many different ways but it does not keep very well. It is one of the least expensive fish.

General nutritional characteristics

Nutritionally, grey mullet is a semi-oily fish (4.9g fat per 100g), extremely rich in proteins (25g per 100g), with fewer calories than lean meat (140 per 100g). It contains lots of omega 3 and vitamin B.

Role in the Dukan Diet

In my diet, this is a fish that really holds its own, especially if bought with care, cooked quickly and grilled with its scales left on, because it is quite filling and slightly chewy. Grey mullet roe is well known as a delicacy. In Provence, it is very much enjoyed eaten as *boutargue* or *poutargue*, which is a paste of dried, salted and pressed mullet roe. You can also use the roe to make your own taramasalata for my diet, by combining some low-fat crème fraîche and oat bran with three drops of olive oil and lemon juice; it must be mixed thoroughly before serving.

How to prepare and eat grey mullet in the Dukan Diet

Grey mullet is best grilled, as this optimizes its slightly fatty meat. It can also be pan-fried, whole and well seasoned. If using larger fish, cutting them up to pan-fry them in smaller pieces is a good idea. Avoid baking this fish in the oven as the flesh will break up.

Grey mullet in chive sauce
Mulet à la sauce ciboulette

1 grey mullet (approx
  350g/12oz)

For the bouillon
1 carrot
1 leek
1 onion
1 bouquet garni
Salt and black pepper

For the sauce
2 tablespoons 3% fat crème
  fraîche
2 tablespoons fat-free fromage
  frais
7–8 fresh chives, chopped
Juice of ½ lemon

Phase 1 PP / Phase 2 PP

Preparation time: 15 minutes
Cooking time: 15 minutes
2 servings

Make a bouillon by placing all the ingredients in a large pan of water.
Bring to the boil and leave to simmer. While the bouillon is simmering,
wash the grey mullet carefully. As soon as the bouillon comes to the boil,
add the fish and leave it to cook, uncovered, for 15 minutes.

Meanwhile, prepare the sauce. Heat the crème fraîche and fromage frais
in a saucepan over a very gentle heat. Add the chives and season with
salt and black pepper.

Once the fish is cooked, remove it from the pan and leave it to cool for a
few minutes. Take the skin off the fish and carefully remove all the flesh
from the bones. Quickly heat the sauce through, pour it over the fish and
serve straightaway.

31. Haddock/smoked haddock

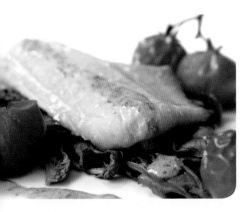

Haddock is a popular white fish that is widely eaten, especially as retailers use it in ready meals, for frozen fish pieces or breaded fish fingers; and of course smoked haddock is also a favourite with many. Most people can still afford to buy fresh haddock and it freezes well.

General nutritional characteristics

As regards nutrition, haddock is the leanest fish known (0.3g fat per 100g) and extremely low in calories. With smoked haddock the calories go up to 101 per 100g, but it is still as lean. Once it is coated in breadcrumbs, however, the calories rocket to 187 and the fat content increases to 9.2g per 100g, introducing in addition 3.1g sugars.

Role in the Dukan Diet

For a long time haddock was considered as a bit of a poor relative because it is so lean; however, being such a low-fat fish means it has lots to offer my diet. Frozen fish fingers are practical for an evening meal, especially Dukan fish fingers. Smoked haddock is a very good slimming food; the smoking process dries the fish so it takes on a different flavour and texture.

How to prepare and eat haddock and smoked haddock in the Dukan Diet

Like cod steaks, haddock can be pan-fried on a bed of chopped onions, browned beforehand. Here is the Dukan fish finger recipe: coat the haddock pieces with oat bran after dipping them in beaten egg. Remember that haddock does not do well in the oven as its flesh is too delicate so it breaks up. Smoked haddock is an absolute treat if you leave it overnight in some milk, then pan-fry it and add a tiny bit of fat-reduced butter. Flaked smoked haddock adds flavour to mixed salads. Finally, smoked haddock is an essential ingredient in a *choucroute de la mer* and it is usually served alongside salmon and some white fish.

Lime-marinated smoked haddock
Haddock mariné au citron vert

600g (1lb 5oz) smoked
  haddock
300ml (10fl oz) skimmed milk
Juice of 4 limes
1 tablespoon soy sauce
1 bunch fresh chives, chopped

Phase 1 PP / Phase 2 PP

Preparation time: 20 minutes
Cooking time: 3 minutes +
  1 hour marinating
4 servings

Poach the smoked haddock for 3 minutes in a mixture of the milk and an equal quantity of boiling water. Then remove the fish and leave it to cool.

Prepare the marinade by combining the lime juice with the soy sauce. Once the fish is cold, remove the skin and cut the flesh into thin strips.

Place the smoked haddock strips in the marinade, mix together and leave in the fridge for at least 1 hour. When ready to serve, sprinkle over the chopped chives.

32. Hake

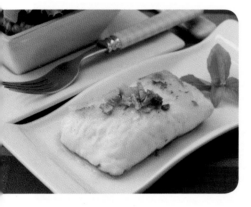

Hake is a fish with fine, white flesh that is much less firm than that of sole or sea bream. Statistically, it seems people enjoy hake more the older they get, which explains why teenagers and young adults often do not think of trying it.

General nutritional characteristics
A lean fish (2g fat per 100g) full of very high-quality proteins (17g per 100g) and very low in calories (92 per 100g).

Role in the Dukan Diet
Great for an adult concerned about their figure and their health. All too often hake is cooked in a court-bouillon, i.e. poached in stock, so it tends to lose its flavour. However, given that hake is a fish with one of the best protein/calorie ratios available, it certainly deserves more attention. Unfortunately, it is not particularly cheap.

How to prepare and eat hake in the Dukan Diet
Leave the fish broth (court-bouillon) alone and try pan-frying instead, as this makes hake far more tasty and appetizing. Also try it in a casserole with some low-fat bacon, onions, garlic, thyme and parsley. Adding a little white wine will not interfere with your dieting, as the alcohol evaporates during cooking. Firmin Arrambide, the Basque chef at the famous Pyrénées restaurant, serves hake roasted with garlic and garnished with clams in their own juices.

Hake and oat bran quiche
Quiche au son et au colin

2 frozen hake steaks, thawed
1 onion, chopped
2 eggs
4 tablespoons oat bran
2 tablespoons wheat bran
2 tablespoons fat-free
  fromage frais
2 tablespoons 3% fat crème
  fraîche

1 teaspoon baking powder
A little fresh dill, to taste
Salt and black pepper

Phase 1 PP / Phase 2 PP

Preparation time: 10 minutes
Cooking time: 35 minutes
2 servings

Preheat the oven to 180°C/350°F/Gas 4.

Once the fish has thoroughly thawed, cut it up into small pieces. Combine the hake pieces with the onion, eggs, oat bran, wheat bran, fromage frais and crème fraîche.

Dissolve the baking powder in a little warm water, add to the hake mixture and stir in well. You can blend the mixture if you prefer. Add the dill, salt and black pepper. Tip into a silicone dish and bake in the oven for 35 minutes.

33. Halibut/smoked halibut

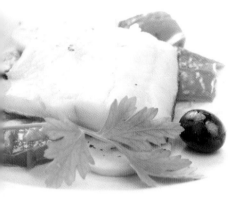

Halibut has chewy white flesh, giving the impression that it comes from an oily fish, whereas in fact it is only semi-oily, which is why it is a very positive food in my diet. Halibut is often served as steaks, which contain very few bones. Smoked halibut is also widely enjoyed.

General nutritional characteristics

Halibut contains slightly more calories than most white fish (96 for steamed halibut and 185 for the smoked version), just as much protein (18g per 100g), but a little more fat (12g per 100g). However, it is a good source of omega 3, vitamin D and selenium.

Role in the Dukan Diet

What makes halibut interesting is its chewy texture far more than its taste, so you will need to add herbs and spices to enhance its flavour rather than mask it.

How to prepare and eat halibut in the Dukan Diet

The best way to cook halibut is to pan-fry it with a few drops of oil wiped away with kitchen paper. *Al dente* courgettes and creamed spinach make wonderful vegetable accompaniments. Try halibut fillets cooked with mussels, chopped shallots and a bouquet garni – and enjoy!

Curried halibut

Flétan au curry

3 shallots, finely chopped
4 tablespoons 3% fat crème
 fraîche
4 tablespoons fat-free fromage
 frais
1 tablespoon curry powder
4 halibut fillets
Salt and black pepper

Phase 1 PP / Phase 2 PP

Preparation time: 15 minutes
Cooking time: 20 minutes
4 servings

Add 2 tablespoons water to a non-stick frying pan and gently cook the shallots.

In a bowl, combine the crème fraîche, fromage frais and curry powder.

Once the shallots have melted down a little, add the halibut fillets to the pan along with the curry powder mixture. Season with salt and black pepper and cook for 15 minutes over a medium heat.

34. Herring

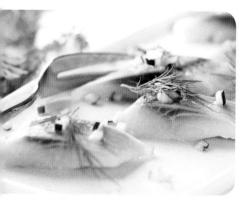

An oily fish that comes in many different forms: fresh, salted and smoked, marinated, as rollmops, fermented Baltic herrings, hot smoked Buckling herrings, kippers, in a sauce or from a tin.

General nutritional characteristics

Along with eel, herring is one of the fattiest and most calorific fish; nevertheless, it still has fewer calories than a rib-eye steak. Herring is extremely rich in omega 3 fatty acids and is a very good food, therefore, for anyone with cardiovascular problems or a tendency to depression. As it is very salty, women who suffer from water retention or cellulite and anyone with high blood pressure should eat it in moderation.

Role in the Dukan Diet

Herring is a great food in my diet because its many guises allow you to ring the changes. Its oily and unctuous flesh is much appreciated and fish oils are the only oils allowed in my diet. Baltic herrings or rollmops make an excellent starter. Smoked herring, bought with its roe and not over-salty, is extremely tasty and certainly does not cost a fortune.

How to prepare and eat herring in the Dukan Diet

Fresh herring works very well cooked in foil, but grilling is a rather unusual and delicious way of preparing it. The best method of baking herrings in the oven is *à la flamande* (Flemish-style): mix the roe with herbs, onions and mustard, then stuff the fish with this mixture and bake it. You can also marinate a fresh herring yourself using lemon juice which slowly pickles the fish.

Dukan rollmop bites
Petites bouchées de rollmop Dukan

10 black peppercorns
2 bay leaves
250ml (9fl oz) cider vinegar
2 teaspoons Dijon mustard
6 herrings in brine
2 cornichons, cut lengthways
  into 6 strips
1 onion, thinly sliced
1 teaspoon fresh dill

1 teaspoon capers

Phase 1 PP / Phase 2 PP

Preparation time: 15 minutes
Cooking time: 20 minutes +
  2 days marinating
2 servings

You will need a large sterilized glass jar and some wooden cocktail sticks.

Add the peppercorns and bay leaves to 100ml (3½oz) water and bring to the boil. Let the water cool down and then pour in the vinegar.

Brush the mustard over the herrings then cover each with cornichon strips, sliced onion, dill and capers.

Carefully roll the herrings up to make rollmops and use cocktail sticks to hold them in place. Put the rollmops in the jar and cover with the vinegar seasoning. Seal the jar and leave to marinate in the fridge for 2 days. When ready to serve, drain the rollmops on some kitchen paper to get rid of any excess liquid.

Handy hint: These rollmops can be served with oat bran blinis (basic recipe: oat bran galette, see page 167) and a fat-free cottage cheese spread seasoned with 2 drops of lemon juice.

35. Mackerel

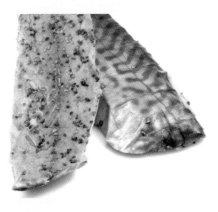

Mackerel is a blue, oily fish, rich in omega 3 and offers protection against heart disease. A cheap fish, available to buy all year round, it can also be purchased tinned.

General nutritional characteristics

Since its oils are of very high quality, mackerel is the fish that offers us the best protection for the heart and the central nervous system as well as providing resistance to stress. This oily fish (17.8g fat per 100g) is a great source of top-quality proteins with hardly any more calories than ordinary beef (128 per 100g for fresh mackerel).

Role in the Dukan Diet

In my diet, mackerel is more commonly eaten tinned than cooked fresh. It makes a very quick and handy snack. Filling and fatty, this is a fish you either love or hate.

How to prepare and eat mackerel in the Dukan Diet

For those of you who do enjoy mackerel, the best way to cook it is grilled with some lemon juice or soy sauce. If it is fatty, the mackerel can easily be baked in the oven with no added fat but stuffed with lots of herbes de Provence. It benefits from being frozen since it is more tender once it has thawed.

Grilled mackerel fillets with fleur de sel

Filets de maquereau grillés à la fleur de sel

4 small mackerel, filleted
Fleur de sel
A little Japanese soy sauce

Phase 1 PP / Phase 2 PP

Preparation time: 10 minutes
Cooking time: 5 minutes
4 servings

Ask your fishmonger to fillet the mackerel.

Score the skin of each fillet. Heat a non-stick frying pan and cook the mackerel, skin side down, for 2–3 minutes until the skin starts to turn crispy. Flip the fillets over and cook the flesh side for 1 minute.

Season with the fleur de sel and drizzle over the soy sauce.

36. Monkfish

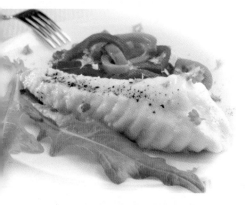

Monkfish has very white, lean, firm, dense, satisfying flesh, without any bones. This is an expensive, luxury fish. It has a slightly sweet taste, a little like lobster or queen scallops. Eating monkfish cheeks is just like eating scallops or crayfish.

General nutritional characteristics

Monkfish is one of the leanest (0.7g fat per 100g) and least calorific (68 calories per 100g) fish in the seas, and it is a good source of proteins with a high nutritional value (15g per 100g).

Role in the Dukan Diet

Monkfish is of prime importance in my diet and I classify it as a 'meat-fish' along with tuna and swordfish because its texture is as firm and chewy as meat. It is this texture which makes monkfish so filling and why you feel so quickly satisfied when eating it.

How to prepare and eat monkfish in the Dukan Diet

Whichever way you cook monkfish, it will taste wonderful. Try it pan-fried with lemon juice and a tablespoon of orange juice; a bigger piece can be baked in the oven, perhaps in foil with some coconut milk (which you discard afterwards); and it also makes terrific kebabs.

Monkfish quiche
Flan de lotte

1.5kg (3lb 5oz) monkfish
4 eggs
250ml (9fl oz) skimmed milk
4 tablespoons 3% fat crème
  fraîche
Salt and black pepper

Phase 1 PP / Phase 2 PP

Preparation time: 10 minutes
Cooking time: 1 hour 15 minutes
4 servings

Cook the monkfish in a court-bouillon (see page 81) for 15 minutes.
Remove the flesh in large pieces.

Preheat the oven to 180°C/400°F/Gas 6.

Make a savoury quiche mixture by combining the eggs, milk and crème
fraîche. Season with salt and black pepper.

Arrange the monkfish pieces in a silicone quiche tin. Pour the quiche
mixture over the fish and press down tightly. Bake in the oven for 1 hour.

Cool, then place in the fridge for 24 hours. Serve with some Dukan
mayonnaise (see page 222) or a light homemade tomato sauce.

37. Plaice

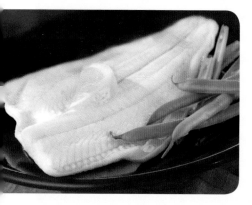

Plaice is a lean flat fish, inexpensive and low in calories. Easily recognizable from its, orange-speckled grey upper side, it is a popular fish, although its flesh is not as firm or delicate as that of sole or turbot. Plaice has a strong iodine taste which some children find off-putting and which can be too strong for people who dislike preparing fish.

General nutritional characteristics

Nutritionally, plaice is as low in calories and fat as any everyday fish that you can buy, which gives it an important place in any diet. It is rich in iron and iodine and recommended, therefore, to anyone suffering from a lazy thyroid or from iron deficiency, such as women with heavy periods who are dieting.

Role in the Dukan Diet

Plaice is an inexpensive, high-quality fish but not one that would be considered as terribly suitable for very special, festive occasions. Its prime interest is for people who really enjoy eating fish but have to watch their pennies too. Plaice also appeals to anyone who loves eating fish products that contain lots of iodine.

How to prepare and eat plaice in the Dukan Diet

Plaice is mostly cooked whole, pan-fried, with its skin left on. Preparing plaice any other way, such as in fillets or in a court-bouillon, risks softening the flesh which can easily disintegrate. A simple recipe is plaice with leeks; or, for an exotic dish and a real treat, try Mauritian-style tomato plaice, prepared with tomato purée, garlic, parsley and ginger.

Stuffed Mediterranean plaice rolls
Paupiettes de carrelet à la méditerranéenne

3 garlic cloves, finely chopped
3 onions, finely chopped
1 x 400g tin chopped tomatoes
1 teaspoon harissa paste
Herbes de Provence
Salt, to taste
1 kg (2lb 4oz) plaice fillets
300g (10½oz) virtually fat-free
    quark or cream cheese (with garlic and herbs)

Phase 2 PV

Preparation time: 25 minutes
Cooking time: 30 minutes
4 servings

Preheat the oven to 180°C/350°F/Gas 4.

Add three drops of oil to a non-stick frying pan and wipe off with kitchen paper. Fry the garlic and onions together and then add the tomatoes. Next, stir in the harissa and herbes de Provence, and season with some salt.

Rinse the plaice fillets, wipe them dry and spread the garlic and herb quark generously over one side. Roll the fillets up and use a wooden cocktail stick to hold each one in place.

Pour the tomato mixture into an ovenproof dish and then add the plaice rolls so that they are roughly three-quarters immersed in the sauce. Bake in the preheated oven for 30 minutes.

38. Pollock/coley

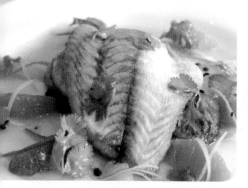

Pollock or coley used to be the poor man's fish that the fishmonger would give to cats. Very lean, with a neutral taste, it benefits from crafty culinary tricks to enhance its flavour. On the plus side, it contains very few bones and is one of the cheapest fish available.

General nutritional characteristics

Nutritionally, pollock or coley is a classic white fish as it is very low in calories (90 per 100g), lean (2g fat per 100g) and full of protein.

Role in the Dukan Diet

In my diet, it is far from being a winner because of its neutral flavour and the fact that it breaks up very easily when cooked. Nevertheless, there are people who champion this fish and know how to make it taste great, so much so that they have even managed to get their children to like it too, and that says it all.

How to prepare and eat pollock or coley in the Dukan Diet

When you cook pollock or coley, you need to take into account how fragile the flesh is. It should be seared, so its surface is sealed and the taste becomes denser. If you bake the fish in the oven stuff it with herbs, garlic and quark. Pollock or coley can also be cooked on a bed of onions, tomatoes and spices. Frozen pieces, once thawed, work well when dipped in beaten egg, then coated in oat bran and gently fried.

Coley fillets with mustard
Filets de lieu noir à la moutarde

2 x 175g (6oz) coley fillets
2 tablespoons 3% fat crème
    traîche
2 tablespoons fat-free fromage
    frais
1 tablespoon mustard
Salt and black pepper

Phase 1 PP / Phase 2 PP

Preparation time: 10 minutes
Cooking time: 30 minutes
2 servings

Preheat the oven to 200°C/400°F/Gas 6. Arrange the coley fillets in an ovenproof dish.

In a bowl, combine the crème fraîche with the fromage frais and mustard and season with salt and black pepper. Pour this mixture over the fish. Reduce the oven temperature to 180°C/350°F/Gas 4, then bake the fillets for 30 minutes.

39. Red mullet

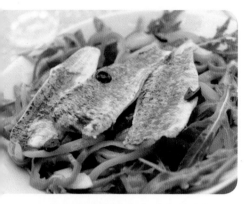

Red mullet is a fish with an unusual flesh and anatomy that people either love or hate. Those who do enjoy eating it really love it. It is a semi-oily fish with a strong taste but it contains a lot of bones, which puts children off, so it tends to be appreciated more by adults.

General nutritional characteristics
Like all fish, red mullet has a lot of protein (20g per 100g) but it also contains 8g of fat along with its omega 3, all for 130 calories per 100g.

Role in the Dukan Diet
For those who like red mullet and never tire of eating it, this is a really useful fish in my diet because you always feel as if you are enjoying a celebratory dish. Semi-oily and very firm, it very quickly makes you feel feel full. Usually it is sold fresh, either whole or in fillets, and you can find three different sizes: baby red mullet, with its very subtle taste and bones you scarcely notice; the traditional medium-sized red mullet; and very large red mullet, which can be baked in the oven and is a magnificent dish, very delicate, sophisticated but expensive.

How to prepare and eat red mullet in the Dukan Diet
How you cook red mullet will depend on the size: small and medium-sized fish can be pan-fried, and larger fish can be baked in the oven with some herbes de Provence, lemon and nothing else. Red mullet is the only fish that can be cooked without it being gutted, which gives it an even stronger flavour. You can also buy frozen fillets.

Red mullet Provençale with aniseed

Rougets anisés à la provençale

4 good-sized red mullet
4 Mediterranean prawns
Pinch of aniseed
1 bay leaf
Fresh thyme
2 tablespoons pastis
Salt and black pepper

Phase 1 PP / Phase 2 PP

Preparation time: 5 minutes
Cooking time: 20 minutes
2 servings

Preheat the oven to 200°C/400°F/Gas 6.

Place the red mullet and prawns on a large square of greaseproof paper. Add the aniseed, bay leaf, thyme and pastis. Season with salt and black pepper and seal up the parcel.

Bake in the oven for 15–20 minutes, until cooked through.

40. Salmon/smoked salmon

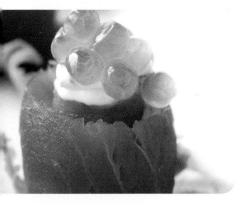

Over the past 20 years salmon has gone from being a luxury food to the most widely sold fish in the world. This change has taken place because salmon is now the most intensively farmed fish, making it available all year round. In practice, the fattier the salmon is, the more enjoyable it is, which means eating the upper part, the part furthest away from the tail.

General nutritional characteristics

As regards nutrition, salmon is an oily fish, but its oils are medicinal and clean out arteries that get clogged up with fat from lamb, pork and rib steak. It is packed with omega 3, and its positive effects on sleep and resistance to stress are beneficial when you are following a weight-loss diet. Lastly, fresh salmon has only 200 calories per 100g and smoked salmon 250 calories – that is around 80 calories per slice. How can you not eat it?

Role in the Dukan Diet

Salmon is one of the main foods in my diet; it is my number one fish. Why? Because, despite its easy availability, you still feel that you are celebrating and eating something special. It is an oily fish that tastes rich and smooth; it has that lovely 'salmony' colour; it is filling, inexpensive and it freezes well without losing any of its taste or texture.

How to prepare and eat salmon in the Dukan Diet

Salmon is a multi-purpose food and can be cooked in every conceivable way: grilled, seared, baked in parcels, steamed, pan-fried, poached, and cooked on a bed of sea salt. Smoked salmon is extremely popular and is found everywhere and in every culture. Marinated salmon has just as many fans too. This all goes to show why it is a top food in my diet.

Salmon and cucumber millefeuille

Millefeuille de concombre et saumon

1 cucumber
2 slices smoked salmon
50g (1¾oz) virtually fat-free
  quark
Salmon or lumpfish roe
Salt and black pepper

Phase 2 PV

Preparation time: 5 minutes
4 servings

Peel the cucumber and cut it into sections approximately 5–8cm (2–3in) long. Then slice each section thinly using a very sharp knife or a vegetable cutter. Cut the smoked salmon slices into pieces the same size as the cucumber.

Make the millefeuille by alternating layers of cucumber, smoked salmon and quark in a loaf tin or terrine, with three to four layers of each. Finish off with a layer of cucumber and garnish with the roe. Season with black pepper to taste. Serve chilled.

41. Sardines

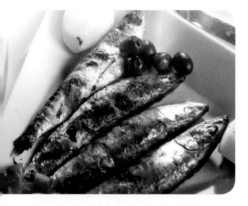

Sardines are small, oily fish and are known across the world as one of the best foods for protecting health. They are especially good for anyone with weight problems, because they are extremely filling.

General nutritional characteristics

Sardine oils are of exceptionally high quality (polyunsaturated) and packed with omega 3. Depending on the season, their fat content varies between 3% and 17% but usually it is 9%, which is less than that of a nice steak (12%). Sardines, especially tinned, are a good source of calcium and are therefore useful for overweight menopausal women.

Role in the Dukan Diet

I consider sardines to be one of the best foods for my diet because they fill you up, they provide fats of exceptional quality, they are inexpensive and come tinned in different sauces – tomato, lemon, oil – as well as in brine.

How to prepare and eat sardines in the Dukan Diet

Sardines can be cooked in many ways and very sophisticated tinned varieties are available if you take the time to select them carefully. Sardines can be grilled, if at all possible on the barbecue, otherwise pan-fry them without any fat. If you cannot bear the smell, oven-bake them in parcels with lemon and coriander. Raw sardines marinate very well: a layer of fish on a layer of garlic, parsley and lemon.

Calabrian-style sardines
Sardines à la calabraise

200g (7oz) tomato passata
3 garlic cloves, crushed
Juice of 1 lemon
12 fresh sardines
Paprika
Salt and black pepper
8 cherry tomatoes, halved
8 quail's eggs, hard-boiled and
   halved

Phase 2 PV

Preparation time: 10 minutes
Cooking time: 12 minutes
2 servings

Pour the passata into a pan, along with the crushed garlic and lemon juice. Cook over a high heat for 5 minutes.

Season the sardines with paprika, salt and black pepper, then gently fry them in a frying pan for 2 minutes. Halfway through, turn them over and, once they are cooked, pour the tomato sauce over the fish.

Finally, add the halved cherry tomatoes and quail's eggs and heat through for a couple of minutes before serving.

42. Sea bream

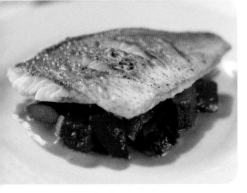

A saltwater fish, the sea bream family includes gilt-head bream, red sea bream and black bream. Bream is one of the best fish for people who are dieting.

General nutritional characteristics

Bream is a good source of proteins (17g per 100g), phosphorus, calcium and iron, yet it is low in fat (2g per 100g) and calories (77 per 100g).

Role in the Dukan Diet

This is a fish with fine, white, dense and filling flesh, a fish for hedonists. It is a very useful food to have in my diet because most people enjoy eating it. Its texture is very firm, its taste is subtle, with a hint of iodine, and it produces a festive-looking dish. Gilt-head bream makes a truly wonderful meal.

How to prepare and eat sea bream in the Dukan Diet

Bream can be cooked as fillets or stuffed with herbs and baked in the oven (gilt-head bream); or if you have a small fish, cook it on a griddle that has been lightly oiled – a few drops only! – then wiped off with kitchen paper. Bream is also very popular for Japanese sashimi. Relatively expensive and appealing to the senses, it is a fish you can put to good strategic use when eating only pure proteins. However, like all white fish, it is less filling than meat. Deep-freezing will impair its flavour but not its nutritional quality.

Sea bream with a red salt crust
Dorade en croûte de sel rouge

1 × 1kg (2lb 4oz) or 2 × 400g
  (14oz) sea bream
1kg (2lb 4oz) sea salt
2 tablespoons tomato purée
Fresh thyme
2 egg whites

Phase 1 PP / Phase 2 PP

Preparation time: 15 minutes
Cooking time: 30 minutes
4 servings

Ask your fishmonger not to de-scale the sea bream and to gut it through its gills so that as little salt as possible gets inside the fish.

Preheat the oven to 200°C/400°F/Gas 6 and line a baking tray with some aluminium foil.

Put the salt and tomato purée in a blender along with the thyme and egg whites and blend very quickly until the salt turns red.

Spread a layer of the salt mixture on the aluminium foil, place the fish on top, then cover entirely with the rest of the salt. Bake in the oven for 30 minutes. Leave to rest for 5 minutes before breaking the salt crust to get to the fish. Use a tablespoon to serve the bream, and be careful to take only the fish and not the salt.

43. Skate

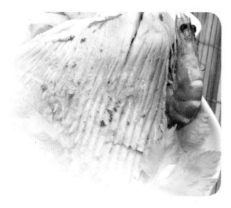

Skate is an impressive fish because its fillets are so thick, it has a cartilaginous bone structure, it is not full of bones and across the fish the texture is crunchy while down the fish it is fibrous. Its two-sided bone structure means you get two fillets of varying thickness, the upper fillet being the more prized.

General nutritional characteristics
Skate is very lean (1g fat per 100g), full of protein (22g per 100g), with only 89 calories per 100g.

Role in the Dukan Diet
In my diet, skate is an extremely useful fish as its flesh is dense, satisfying, packed with proteins and ultra-lean. Unfortunately, though, its slight aroma of ammonia means that people tend either to love it or hate it. Washing the fish under lots of cold water gets rid of this ammonia smell.

How to prepare and eat skate in the Dukan Diet
Traditionally, skate is poached, then covered with *beurre noisette*, brown butter, with lemon juice and parsley. For my diet, the butter is replaced by using a small brush to brush the fish with some walnut oil for at least one minute, then adding capers and lemon juice so that you have the taste of the walnuts but without the calories.

Skate wing with herbs and capers

Aile de raie aux fines herbes et aux câpres

1 fairly thick skate wing
1 large bunch of fresh mixed
   herbs (e.g. chives, parsley,
   tarragon)
Salt and black pepper
½ glass white wine vinegar
1 lemon, cut in half

1 tablespoon capers

Phase 1 PP / Phase 2 PP

Preparation time: 25 minutes
Cooking time in pressure cooker:
  5 minutes
2 servings

Wash the skate wing in plenty of water. Chop 1 tablespoon of the herbs and reserve. Using a pressure cooker, place the skate in a perforated steaming pan insert on top of a bed of the remaining herbs. Season with salt and black pepper and sprinkle over a few more herbs.

Mix the vinegar with 1½ glasses water and pour this mixture into the pressure cooker. Place the insert in an upper position. Close the pressure cooker and cook for 5 minutes from when the pressure starts.

Once the skate is cooked, remove the herbs and the skin. Take the upper part of the skate off the bone and place on a warmed plate. Do the same with the bottom part of the wing.

Serve the fish piping hot. Squeeze over the juice of one lemon half, sprinkle with the reserved chopped herbs and the capers, and garnish with the remaining lemon cut into quarters.

44. Swordfish

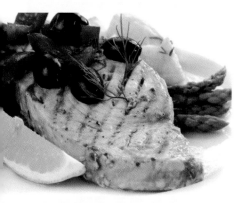

A semi-oily saltwater fish, easily recognizable because of its sword-shaped mouth and crescent-shaped tail, and , in the case of certain legendary species, for the way it spreads its dorsal fin like a sail.

General nutritional characteristics

Swordfish is high in protein (19g per 100g) and iron and has an average fat content of 4.5g per 100g. Recommended for anyone at risk of cardiovascular disease who wants some protective fish oils.

Role in the Dukan Diet

Swordfish meat is both delicate and compact and leaves you feeling nicely satisfied. It has a special place in the Dukan Diet as its flesh is not as moist as that of tuna and it is not as fatty as salmon.

How to prepare and eat swordfish in the Dukan Diet

Cut your swordfish into slices and either grill or pan-fry them. Or make kebabs, alternating the swordfish with prawns and scallops, or try it as a carpaccio, marinated in lime juice.

Swordfish carpaccio with dried peppers and tomatoes

Carpaccio d'espadon aux poivrons et tomates séchés

350g (12oz) swordfish
85g (3oz) roasted peppers
 in oil
85g (3oz) dried tomatoes in oil
Juice of 4 lemons
1 tablespoon chopped
 fresh parsley
Salt and black pepper

Phase 2 PV

Preparation time: 15 minutes +
 30 minutes freezing
Marinating time: 20 minutes
4 servings

Clean the swordfish and remove the skin and central bone. Wash and dry it, then leave to harden in the freezer for 30 minutes so that it is easier to cut up. Remove from the freezer and slice as thinly as possible.

Lay the slices in a fairly deep dish. Wipe any oil off the dried peppers and tomatoes, then chop them up into small pieces. Scatter them over the fish. Pour the lemon juice over the carpaccio, add the chopped parsley and season with salt and black pepper.

Cover with clingfilm and leave to marinate in the fridge for at least 20 minutes.

45. Trout (rainbow and salmon)

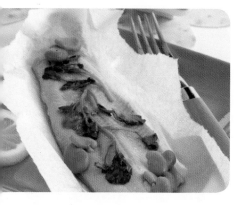

Trout contains a lot of proteins and few calories, but it is also an attractive fish; rainbow trout flesh in particular has a lovely colour. Trout is easy to farm, which means it is affordable and widely available.

General nutritional characteristics

Trout is a fish that could easily get overlooked but it is actually almost as nutritionally valuable as salmon. However, trout is a little less oily, which means it does not taste quite so rich. It has slightly less omega 3, but it contains fewer calories and more protein.

Role in the Dukan Diet

Trout is an ideal fish for the Dukan method because it is semi-oily and rich in omega 3. It is rich in proteins with an excellent nutritional value. You can also vary the flavour by alternating between rainbow trout and salmon trout.

How to prepare and eat trout in the Dukan Diet

The standard, traditional recipe is trout with almonds. You can still include this in the diet by cooking the fish in lots of sliced almonds, so that the trout absorbs all the flavour from the nuts. Then, when you are about to serve, remove all the almonds while ensuring that the fish remains hot. Trout lends itself to a whole range of recipes, and those particularly suitable for my diet include trout mousse (made with milk and eggs), smoked trout millefeuille and trout on a bed of leeks.

Baked trout parcels
Papillotes de truite

4 trout, cleaned and gutted
2 garlic cloves, finely chopped
2 sprigs fresh basil, finely
   chopped
2 onions, diced
Salt and black pepper

Phase 1 PP / Phase 2 PP

Preparation time: 20 minutes
Cooking time: 15 minutes
4 servings

First make the stuffing by mixing together the garlic, basil and onions, and season with salt and black pepper.

Fill each trout with this mixture and wrap them individually in a sheet of greaseproof paper, then again in some aluminium foil.

Cook the fish for about 15 minutes either on the barbecue or in a medium oven (200°C/400°F/Gas 6).

46. Tuna

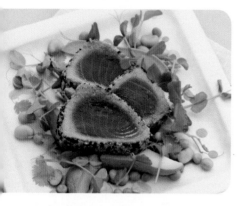

Tuna is a thoroughly modern food, available the world over now that these big fish are caught using sophisticated fishing fleets. It is very nutritious and hugely popular with the general public, especially as it is available tinned and in different sauces.

General nutritional characteristics

Nutritionally, tuna is the fish that contains the most protein (26.5g per 100g); it has far less fat than people think (1.7g per 100g in brine, and 6g when raw) and far fewer calories than an ordinary steak (150 per 100g). What is more, tuna contains as much iron as red meat and has an exceptional amount of vitamin PP, which helps with energy production and to keep the nervous system working properly.

Role in the Dukan Diet

Tuna is a key food in my diet. Of all fish it has the most protein. It is the most filling, its meat is the firmest and it can be cooked in so many different ways. Tinned in brine, it is (along with crab sticks) the fish most commonly used by my patients and people who follow my diet.

How to prepare and eat tuna in the Dukan Diet

There are lots of ways to prepare it. A grilled tuna steak is a magnificent way to serve this fish. Take care not to overcook it, as this will dry it out and its tasty juices will evaporate. Also avoid pricking it while it is cooking. You can cook tuna in the oven and in parcels but then it will lose much of its flavour. Another fantastic way of eating tuna is raw, as tuna tartare or carpaccio. Tahitian-style tuna – small cubes marinated in lime – will melt in your mouth, full of flavour. However, do take care if you are buying tuna to eat raw: contaminated tuna, unlike all other fish, cannot be detected by its smell, its taste or even a change in texture. So it has to be eaten absolutely fresh and, if you have the slightest doubt, cook it as this will eliminate any possible risk.

Tuna loaf
Cake au thon

2 eggs
40g (1½oz) virtually fat-free
  quark
40g (1½oz) fat-free fromage
  frais
1 × 185g tin tuna, in spring
  water or brine
1 teaspoon curry powder

4 tablespoons skimmed milk
Salt and black pepper

Phase 1 PP / Phase 2 PP

Preparation time: 8 minutes
Cooking time: 40 minutes
2 servings

Preheat the oven to 230°C/450°F/Gas 8.

Mix all the ingredients together until you have a smooth and even
mixture, and pour into a loaf tin. Bake in the oven for 30 minutes, then
reduce the temperature to 180°C/350°F/Gas 4 and cook
for a further 10 minutes.

The loaf is ready when it has turned golden brown.

47. Turbot

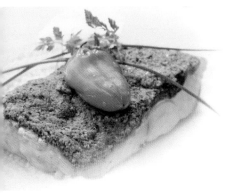

Turbot is rare, delicate and expensive – a fish often found on menus in the best, chic restaurants. However, it is also a fish that offers many rewards; a person who is dieting will feast for a long time on the memory of a lovely, thick fillet of turbot.

General nutritional characteristics

As far as nutrition goes, forget about the calories (116 per 100g), its proteins and its fats. Just enjoy and don't count!

Role in the Dukan Diet

In my diet, turbot is too much of a luxury food to feature on a dieter's everyday menu, which is a pity because it is as delicious as it is lean. Set yourself a goal: when you are halfway to achieving your target weight, and then again once you attain it, treat yourself to a nice piece of turbot either poached or baked in the oven – that is if you like fish, of course!

How to prepare and eat turbot in the Dukan Diet

Make sure you cook your turbot to best advantage; you can serve it with shellfish, Dublin Bay prawns and a bisque, and chanterelle mushrooms. But whatever you do, try not to overcook it as that would be disastrous.

Vanilla-flavoured turbot
Turbot à la vanille

4 tablespoons 3% fat crème
  fraîche
1 vanilla pod
1 teaspoon dried thyme,
  crumbled up
2 teaspoons soy sauce
Juice of ½ lemon
4 200g (7oz) turbot fillets

Salt and black pepper
1 tablespoon chopped fresh
  chives

Phase 1 PP / Phase 2 PP

Preparation time: 15 minutes
Cooking time: 10 minutes
4 servings

Put the crème fraîche in a small pan and scrape in the vanilla seeds from the pod. Add the thyme, 1 teaspoon of the soy sauce and the lemon juice. Leave the mixture to rest.

Heat a non-stick frying pan, add 1 tablespoon water with the remaining soy sauce and sear the turbot.

Season with salt and black pepper. Cook the turbot for 8–10 minutes, turning the fillets over regularly so that they cook through and change colour slightly.

Over a gentle heat, warm the sauce mixture and serve with the fish. Garnish with the chopped chives.

48. Whiting

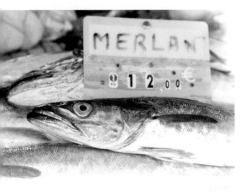

Whiting is a fish with lean, white flesh and a soft texture; it is easily digestible and reasonably priced but not hugely popular.

General nutritional characteristics
Whiting is a lean fish (0.5g fat per 100g), a good source of proteins (15g per 100g) and low in calories (70 per 100g).

Role in the Dukan Diet
Whiting is not a star of the seas in my diet because it needs careful cooking for its true flavour to be brought out. It is usually fried or cooked in breadcrumbs and is less appealing when either poached or baked in foil. It is more enjoyable to eat when used as an ingredient in fish fingers and flaked fish.

How to prepare and eat whiting in the Dukan Diet
Some people happily grill whiting as they do not mind it falling apart when it is cooked. A good way to use it is in a fish soup or in stuffing.

Whiting gratin
Gratin de merlan

200g (7oz) button
mushrooms, sliced
3 tablespoons balsamic
vinegar
Fresh parsley, chopped
1 shallot, finely chopped
Salt and black pepper
2 whiting fillets
1 egg

3 tablespoons 3% fat crème
fraîche
30g (1oz) low-fat Gruyère
cheese, grated

Phase 2 PV

Preparation time: 10 minutes
Cooking time: 15 minutes
2 servings

Preheat the oven to 200°C/400°F/Gas 6.

In a well-heated frying pan, fry the mushrooms in the balsamic vinegar for 5 minutes. Add the parsley, shallot, salt and black pepper and stir together well.

Cut the whiting fillets into large pieces and place them in a gratin dish. Pour over the mushroom and shallot mixture.

In a small bowl, combine the egg with the crème fraîche and pour over the fish. Sprinkle with the grated Gruyère and bake in the oven for 15 minutes. Serve piping hot.

49. Calamari/squid

Calamari is a healthy and extremely lean food, packed with protein, low in calories and naturally suited to a slimming programme.

General nutritional characteristics

When it comes to nutrition, it would seem that calamari was created specially for my diet: 87 calories, 16g protein and 1.4g fat per 100g. However, if you fry the calamari, it loses its gastronomic interest as well as any nutritional value.

Role in the Dukan Diet

In my diet, calamari has the advantage of being one of the most substantial and firm blocks of proteins there is and it requires a lot of chewing. Calamari takes a long time to digest, which means you feel full for longer. Lastly, if you know how to cook calamari properly, it is a subtle and flavoursome food. On top of this, it freezes well and is a little out of the ordinary so it becomes a real treat from the seas.

How to prepare and eat calamari in the Dukan Diet

Calamari can be used in a whole range of different recipes, but the best way by far is to cook it on a griddle pan, with three drops of oil wiped away with kitchen paper, on a bed of onions, tomatoes and strips of fish. There are two types of calamari: the larger calamari which are better 'endowed' in body than in tentacles, and the smaller mini calamari that also work very well on the griddle.

Calamari Provençale
Calamar à la provençale

For the tomato sauce
1 × 400g tin chopped tomatoes
1 garlic clove, chopped
1 onion, chopped
1 shallot, chopped
A little fresh parsley
1 sprig of fresh thyme
1 bay leaf
Salt and black pepper

For the calamari
1 squid, cleaned and cut into
    medium-sized strips
2 onions, chopped
Fish stock, with fat removed

Phase 2 PV

Preparation time: 20 minutes
Cooking time: 1 hour
4 servings

Make a tomato sauce by mixing together all the ingredients.

In a non-stick frying pan, fry the squid and chopped onions in the fat-free fish stock. Transfer to a casserole, cover with the tomato sauce and cook gently over a low heat for 1 hour.

50. Clams

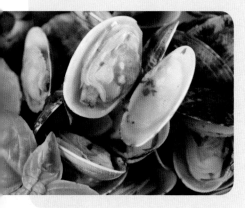

Round, striated shellfish that live in sandy areas, clams are harvested from the sea, then kept in pools until they reach maturity. When you buy clams make sure they are closed tight, wash them thoroughly to get rid of any sand and eat them as soon as they open up.

General nutritional characteristics

As far as nutrition is concerned, clams are one of the fattiest shellfish (10g per 100g), but this is because they contain fatty acids that are good for the heart. They are a little high in calories, but eating them slowly means you concentrate on their flavour and texture, and like all seafood they are full of proteins with a good nutritional value.

Role in the Dukan Diet

In my diet, clams will appeal to those who enjoy something a little exotic. Moreover, because of their high protein content, they are very filling. The fish oils clams contain give them a creamy flavour, and they can be used to good effect, proving that following a weight-loss diet does not mean you have to restrict your choices. Use them, for example, to transform a soup into an extraordinary dish that will delight your guests.

How to prepare and eat clams in the Dukan Diet

Clams can be eaten raw as long as you ensure that they are fresh and free of all sand. If you are cooking them, try stuffed clams, for which there are many different variations. You could, for instance, stuff them with tiny vegetables. I especially like clams cooked to a recipe called 'Kari Gosse' – originally a sailors' dish, it uses a wonderful blend of rare curry spices given an extra kick by our own French Espelette chilli peppers. Chef Rick Stein also has a spicy clam masala dish you could adapt for the diet.

Seafood stew
Pot-au-feu de fruits de mer

1 bouquet garni	4 shallots (left whole)	**Phase 2 PV**
1 teaspoon ground coriander	500g (1lb 2oz) mussels	
1 pinch nutmeg	500g (1lb 2oz) cockles	**Preparation time : 35 minutes**
Salt and black peppercorns	500g (1lb 2oz) clams	**Cooking time : 1 hour 15 minutes**
6 carrots, peeled and chopped		**4 servings**
2 turnips, diced		
2 fennel bulbs, quartered		
2 leeks, sliced		
1 stick celery, chopped		

Bring 2.5 litres (4¼ pints) of water to the boil in a large pan. Add the bouquet garni, coriander, nutmeg and a teaspoon of black peppercorns.

Put the carrots and turnips into the stock and cook, covered, for 30 minutes. Then add the remaining vegetables and cook for a further 30 minutes.

Scrub all the shellfish under cold water and remove the beards from the mussels. Use a slotted spoon to take the vegetables out of the stock and divide them among four individual bowls. Add the shellfish to the stock and cook until they open, about 1 minute. Remove the shellfish, discarding any that have refused to open, and arrange over the vegetables.

Strain the stock and shellfish juice through a conical strainer, adjust the seasoning and pour the broth into the bowls. Serve immediately.

51. Cockles

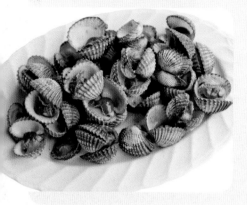

An edible, little, rounded shellfish that contains a small white cockle, meaty and quite firm in texture, with a tiny bump of orange coral. In France, cockles from Normandy are fuller and more sought-after than the ones from Brittany.

General nutritional characteristics

Nutritionally, cockles seem to have been specially designed for my diet: they taste good, are unusual, have very few calories (47 per 100g) and plenty of proteins, and they are very reasonably priced.

Role in the Dukan Diet

Cockles offer a nice but occasional contribution to my diet. Worth keeping in mind for the useful variety they offer, especially if your diet is stagnating, as they contain iodine. They are very lean, full of proteins, but low in calories; however, they take some time to rinse, to remove all the sand, and cook.

How to prepare and eat cockles in the Dukan Diet

Cook them in a stew pot and keep turning them over and over to get rid of any last remaining grains of sand. Once cooked, they can be shelled and used in different and sophisticated ways; for example, if you cook them very gently in a tamarind and coriander sauce, these humble little shellfish will be transformed into a dish fit for a king.

Curried cockles
Coques au curry

2 litres (3½ pints) cockles
100ml (3½fl oz) white wine
2 shallots, thinly sliced
1 tablespoon curry powder
1 bunch fresh coriander, finely
  chopped
200ml (7fl oz) 3% fat single
  cream

Phase 1 PP / Phase 2 PP

Preparation time: 30 minutes
Cooking time: 15 minutes
6 servings

Scrub and wash the cockles. Cook them in a large flameproof casserole over a high heat for 10 minutes with the white wine and 100ml (3½fl oz) water. Stir them around from time to time. They are cooked once the shells have opened. Remove the cockles from the shells and keep them warm.

In a non-stick, deep-sided frying pan, gently brown the shallots in 2 tablespoons water. Next add the curry powder, half the bunch of finely chopped coriander and the low-fat single cream. Reduce over a low heat for 5 minutes. Then add the cockles.

Combine all the ingredients carefully and pour into individual dishes, sprinkle over the remaining coriander and serve immediately.

52. Crab

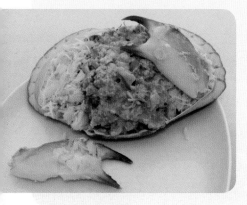

The white meat of crab is beautiful and festive with a wonderful delicate flavour; the only drawback is the price and worries about cholesterol, which, if you avoid the coral, are unfounded.

General nutritional characteristics
As far as nutrition goes, it is difficult to find a leaner food (2g fat per 100g), with more protein (20g per 100g) and fewer calories (100 per 100g).

Role in the Dukan Diet
Crab is a great asset to my diet: it is as distinctive as it is full of proteins of excellent nutritional value, as low in fat as it is tasty, and as sophisticated and filling as crayfish, especially if you go for Chatka crab which is the best in the world.

How to prepare and eat crab in the Dukan Diet
Crab is easy to prepare; it teams up like a dream with Dukan mayonnaise (see page 222), and together they provide a truly wonderful gourmet experience. If your weight is stagnating or you are finding yourself getting stuck in a rut, crab will give you a boost as it offers such pleasure while making your diet work.

Crab balls
Boulettes de crabe

500g (1lb 2oz) flaked crab meat
3 tablespoons cornflour
Juice of ½ lemon
2 tablespoons ground cumin
2 tablespoons finely chopped fresh coriander
1 teaspoon ground turmeric

2 tablespoons ground ginger
1 egg yolk, beaten

Phase 1 PP / Phase 2 PP

Preparation time: 2 minutes +
1 hour resting
Cooking time: 5 minutes
4 servings

Mix together all the ingredients except the egg yolk. Leave the mixture to rest for 1 hour, then form into little balls.

Preheat the oven to 180°C/350°F/Gas 4.

Place the crab balls in an ovenproof dish, brush with the beaten egg yolk and cook in the oven for 5 minutes.

53. Crayfish/crawfish

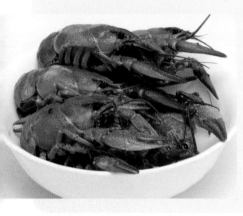

This is a luxury, celebration food like lobster and has a place in a slimming diet only because it opens up the horizon if you are growing bored, your weight is stagnating or if you need a little reward or pleasure.

General nutritional characteristics

As far as nutrition goes, crayfish/crawfish is lean (1.5g fat per 100g), high in protein (18g per 100g) and very low in calories (90 per 100g), but unfortunately its steep price limits its usefulness.

Role in the Dukan Diet

Crayfish ought to be the ideal food in my diet since it combines all the qualities we are looking for: it is lean, stuffed with high-quality proteins, low in calories, delicious and with a texture that is dense and extremely filling. However, including it as a food that you can eat as much as you want is not easy for those who cannot afford to treat themselves to it. Nevertheless, crayfish/crawfish makes an occasional treat and it can be bought live or already prepared, or even frozen (but the fish must be frozen live). As a rule, you need 800g (just under 2lb) to serve two people. Frozen crayfish does not taste quite as good as fresh.

How to prepare and eat crayfish in the Dukan Diet

The traditional way to serve crayfish is cooked in a court-bouillon, but do not cook it for longer than 10 minutes or it will become rubbery. Then eat it cold with mayonnaise – try my Dukan mayonnaise on page 222 so that you avoid fats when on my diet. It can also be grilled and covered with a sauce made from chives, shallots, oregano, garlic, parsley, chilli and lemon juice.

Stir-fried crayfish tails and prawns
Crevettes et queues de langouste au wok

20 shelled, raw prawns
1 small fennel bulb, chopped
1 red pepper, chopped
20 crayfish tails
150g (5½oz) fat-free yoghurt
Pinch of cayenne pepper
Salt and black pepper

Phase 2 PV

Preparation time: 15 minutes
Cooking time: 10 minutes
2 servings

Lightly oil the wok, then wipe with some kitchen paper and gently fry the prawns. Add the fennel and red pepper and fry gently for a few minutes. Add the crayfish tails and leave to simmer gently for a few more minutes.

Stir in the yoghurt and cayenne pepper and season with a little salt and black pepper. Serve immediately in ramekin dishes.

54. Dublin Bay prawns

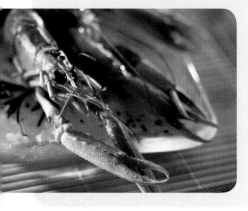

Fun, festive, colourful, a little luxurious and the very opposite of what we traditionally imagine diet food to be. All the same, these prawns are costly and should be kept in reserve for times when dieting gets tough and you need cheering up.

General nutritional characteristics

Nutritionally, Dublin Bay prawns have everything going for them. As well as tasting great and filling you up, they are lean (1g fat per 100g), rich in good proteins (17g per 100g) and contain only 91 calories per 100g.

Role in the Dukan Diet

If you like Dublin Bay prawns and you can afford them, go ahead and enjoy them in my diet; they are delicious and subtle, lean and low in calories, and, most important, I give them a place in my 'slow foods' family – shelling the prawns takes time which makes you slow down and enjoy their flavour. Lastly, they have a good texture and are filling; as they take some time to digest, you will remain satiated for longer.

How to prepare and eat Dublin Bay prawns in the Dukan Diet

These prawns are prepared in a very traditional way – cooked in a court-bouillon to which you should add a little white wine, carrots, onion and a bouquet garni. Be careful not to overcook them or the flavour will be impaired: three minutes for small Dublin Bay prawns and seven for the larger ones. While on the subject of size, the large ones are much more expensive than the little ones, which actually taste better. A few shelled Dublin Bay prawns add colour and protein to a lamb's lettuce salad.

Dublin Bay prawn gratin
Gratin de langoustines

12 raw Dublin Bay prawns
2 shallots, finely chopped
4 tomatoes, skinned, deseeded
  and chopped
1 bouquet garni
Salt and black pepper
100ml (3½fl oz) dry white wine
Cognac flavouring (www.
  mydukandietshop.co.uk)

2 tablespoons 3% fat crème
  fraîche

Phase 2 PV

Preparation time: 15 minutes
Cooking time: 20 minutes
2 servings

Preheat the oven to 150°C/300°F/Gas 2.

Cook the prawns in a court-bouillon (see page 81) for 5 minutes. Shell them and divide between two individual gratin dishes.

Soften the shallots in a little water in a pan. Add the tomatoes and the bouquet garni. Season with a little salt and black pepper.

Add the dry white wine, and 100ml (3½fl oz) water mixed with the cognac flavouring. Leave to simmer for 10 minutes.

Add the low-fat crème fraîche, pour the sauce over the Dublin Bay prawns and bake in the oven for 10 minutes.

55. Lobster

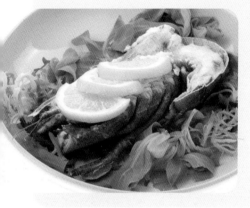

A luxury food for special occasions, lobster features only now and then in a slimming diet, to help you tackle stagnation or to give yourself a treat.

General nutritional characteristics
Lobster is lean (1g fat per 100g), high in protein (20g per 100g) and very low in calories (91 per 100g), but does any of this count when lobster is such an expensive food? If you are not put off by the cost, it is one of the foods with the highest vitamin B12 content; it can now also be bought frozen at a more reasonable price from supermarkets.

Role in the Dukan Diet
Being so low in fat and calories and so high in proteins, lobster would be the dream food for my diet, but to overlook its cost would be an affront to all those people who simply cannot afford it. If you are splashing out for major celebrations, just remember that you can buy lobster live or frozen (but it must have been a living animal that was frozen), that the meat is only 30% of the total weight, and that the female is fuller than the male and its flesh is said to be better than that of the male.

How to prepare and eat lobster in the Dukan Diet
Traditionally a lobster is poached; serve it with some Dukan mayonnaise (see page 222). However, it can also be cooked in the oven, cut into two and placed quickly under the grill, or braised *à l'américaine* in a garlic, shallot and tomato sauce which also uses the lobster's coral. Do be careful not to overcook lobster, otherwise it will lose its melt-in-the-mouth texture and become stringy and rubbery.

Lobster medallions in aspic
Médaillons de homard en gelée

1 × 25g sachet aspic jelly
1 bunch of white asparagus
1 cooked, frozen lobster
3 hard-boiled eggs, halved
3 slices smoked salmon
A little fresh flat-leaf parsley,
  chopped

Phase 2 PV

Preparation time: 20 minutes
Cooking time: 30 minutes +
  2 hours chilling
6 servings

Make up the aspic jelly by following the instructions on the packet.

Cook the asparagus and leave to cool on a clean tea towel so that all the water is soaked up.

Cut the lobster into medallions and arrange them in a small dish. Cover with the egg halves and pour over the aspic mixture. Refrigerate for at least 2 hours.

When ready to serve, turn the lobster aspic out on to a serving dish and arrange the asparagus around it, along with the smoked salmon slices cut in half. Lastly, to add a little colour, sprinkle over the chopped parsley.

56. Mussels

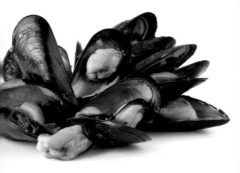

An extremely useful food, from both a nutritional and a gastronomic point of view, and very inexpensive as seafood proteins go. The only drawback is that mussels constantly filter the surrounding sea water, picking up and harbouring everything in it, so you need to take great care when buying and storing them.

General nutritional characteristics

We already know that, as far as nutrition goes, mussels are ideal. See for yourself: 66 calories, 12g protein and 2g fat per 100g. Their price is just as attractive too.

Role in the Dukan Diet

Mussels are a dream food in my diet as they are stuffed with proteins and even more so with iron, containing more than meat (note that half the female population is deficient in iron). Mussels are lean with very few calories. Moreover, they also belong to my 'slow-foods' category, their shells making them slow to eat and forcing voracious eaters to slow down – those who would otherwise gulp their food without giving their brains time to produce a feeling of satiety. Try to eat them as often as possible by cooking them in lots of different ways.

How to prepare and eat mussels in the Dukan Diet

A traditional dish is *moules marinières*, mussels cooked in white wine – the alcohol evaporates during cooking – with plenty of onions and garlic that melts in the mouth, having lost its odour from being cooked. Shelled and added to a salad, mussels make a great lunch to take to work. You can also cook them in a cream sauce, using fat-reduced cream. Finally, after you have removed the mussels from their shells, try pan-frying them before adding them to an omelette – absolutely delicious!

Normandy-style mussels in cream
Moules normandes à la crème

1kg (2lb 4oz) small mussels, cleaned
2 tablespoons cider vinegar
4 leeks, white part only, cooked and cut into small chunks
1 carrot, cooked and thinly sliced

2 shallots, finely chopped
2 tablespoons 3% fat cream

Phase 2 PV

Preparation time: 5 minutes
Cooking time: 10–20 minutes
2 servings

Place the mussels in a large pan and half-cover with water. Pour in the cider vinegar and add the leeks, carrot and shallots. Stir from time to time until all the mussels have opened up (discard any that refuse to open). Once the mussels have opened, add the low-fat cream, stir well and serve.

57. Prawns/shrimps

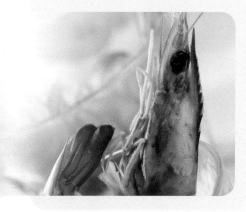

Prawns/shrimps are a cornerstone of any slimming programme and in particular of a protein-rich diet where quantity is unrestricted, and most especially if you are looking for diversity, pleasure, texture and colour.

General nutritional characteristics
Like most other shellfish, prawns are packed with protein and contain little fat or calories. If cholesterol is an issue, you do not have to ban prawns from your table as the only parts to avoid are the head and coral.

Role in the Dukan Diet
In my diet prawns are a top-notch food, available these days to everyone as a result of improvements in fishing techniques, large-scale breeding, trading between countries and the availability now of other types that live in oceans and waters further away (northern prawns found in the deep waters around Norway, Mediterranean gambas, bouquet prawns, pink shrimps from Senegal, etc.). Along with eggs, tuna in brine and chicken liver, prawns are one of the most filling foods in the world. What is more, they are a 'slow food', taking time to shell. Lastly, prawns are firm and substantial; they take ages to digest but have an exquisite flavour and texture.

How to prepare and eat prawns in the Dukan Diet
Prawns are used in all cultures and can be prepared in so many different ways. You can buy them frozen and shelled. Try to avoid very small, shelled, frozen prawns that, when thawed, give out a lot of water, which leaves them tasting rubbery and wishy-washy. Traditionally, prawns are pan-fried in garlic or served with a fat-free mayonnaise, but they appear in all sorts of mixed salads, kebabs and omelettes. For a slightly more sophisticated twist, try them served Creole-style or with artichoke hearts or in a Thai coconut milk curry.

Sautéed ginger prawns
Gambas sautées au gingembre

1 piece (5cm/2inch) fresh
  ginger
4 small onions, finely chopped
8 large raw Mediterranean
  prawns
1 low-salt fish stock cube,
  dissolved in 200ml (7fl oz)
  water
Salt and black pepper

Phase 1 PP / Phase 2 PP

Preparation time: 5 minutes
Cooking time: 15 minutes
2 servings

Peel the ginger and use a vegetable peeler to cut it into very thin slices.

Warm a non-stick frying pan and add 2 tablespoons water. When the water is hot, add the onions and ginger to make a nice bed for the Mediterranean prawns. Place the prawns on the bed of onions and ginger and pour over the fish stock. Cook for about 15 minutes.

Season with salt and black pepper and serve.

58. Oysters

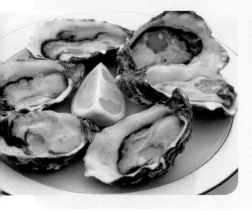

In any diet, oysters are an invaluable food as they offer luxury, celebration and variety at a price that remains affordable if you shop wisely (that is directly from the producer).

General nutritional characteristics

As far as nutrition is concerned, oysters are lean whatever the variety. They have 2–5g carbohydrates and only 65 calories per 100g. But they are packed with iron (three times more than red meat) and a whole array of rare vitamins and trace elements such as copper, selenium and zinc. However, like mussels, oysters spend their time filtering sea water and so they pick up some of its pollutants, in particular the hepatitis virus.

Role in the Dukan Diet

In my diet, oysters are a great support, being a lean food that is full of protein and low in calories but with a little extravagance. They also have to be eaten slowly and with some ceremony, and they are extremely filling. Finally, oysters offer you the chance to ring the changes as they are a food group with plenty of variety: each sort has its own special flavour and texture, so discover which your own particular favourite is!

How to prepare and eat oysters in the Dukan Diet

As a rule oysters are eaten raw with a drizzle of lemon juice; however, they can also be used in cooked dishes. An oat bran galette makes a good accompaniment. Be careful never to place an oyster on ice as it will lose its flavour.

Oyster gratin
Gratin d'huîtres

3 dozen oysters
1 onion, studded with 2 cloves
1 carrot, sliced
1 bouquet garni
100ml (3½fl oz) white wine
2 tablespoons cornflour
100ml (3½fl oz) skimmed
  milk
Salt and black pepper

A little low-fat Emmental
  cheese, grated (optional)

Phase 2 PV

Preparation time: 15 minutes
Cooking time: 30 minutes
4 servings

Prepare the stock: put the oysters, onion, carrot, bouquet garni, white wine and 100ml (3½fl oz) water in a saucepan and leave to cook for 20 minutes.

Preheat the oven to 220°C/425°F/Gas 7.

Make the béchamel sauce. Put the cornflour in a pan and gradually blend in the milk. Cook for a few minutes over a low heat, stirring continuously as the sauce thickens, then season with salt and black pepper.

Open up the oysters and arrange them in an ovenproof dish. Pour the hot sauce on to each and every oyster and sprinkle over the grated cheese (if using). Bake in the oven for 2 minutes, then serve immediately.

59. Scallops

A luxury food, expensive but very tasty, scallops are both lean and high in proteins and iodine.

General nutritional characteristics
Scallops are blocks of proteins with great nutritional values as they contain hardly any fat (0.8g per 100g – so really lean) and 2.4g carbohydrates, which gives them a slightly caramelized taste when cooked. Scallops are also very rich in B12, a rare vitamin mostly found in animal meat.

Role in the Dukan Diet
Exactly the sort of food that is universally popular, scallops have to remain a very occasional treat because of their cost. If you are happy to eat frozen scallops and take a little time to prepare them carefully, they are half the price and can become one of those foods eaten once or twice a week in my diet to add a little fun, variety and pleasure. Scallops are a real comfort food because of their texture and their sugars, which caramelize during cooking. Here is a useful tip: thaw your frozen scallops in some milk for at least a day and they will taste as tender as fresh scallops.

How to prepare and eat scallops in the Dukan Diet
Traditionally, scallops are lightly fried after the ritual 'three drops of oil plus kitchen paper' routine. Do be careful, though, because if you overcook them for just one minute, their magical texture will be ruined. Always remember that less is more, as scallops can even be eaten raw or as a tartare. If you buy them frozen, check carefully to see that they are not the smaller, farmed queen scallops, which are not so flavoursome. In France, the very best scallops are called *la Normande* and have their own quality label. If you buy 6.5kg (14lb 5oz) of scallops in their shells, you will end up with 1kg (2lb 4oz) of scallops to eat.

Scallop bake
Cassolette de Saint-Jacques

2 medium onions, thinly sliced
2 medium shallots, thinly
sliced
100ml (3½fl oz) dry white wine
100ml (3½fl oz) 3% fat crème
fraîche
400g (14oz) small frozen
scallops, thawed

250g (9oz) small frozen raw
prawns, thawed
250g (9oz) frozen mussels,
thawed

Phase 2 PV

Preparation time: 10 minutes
Cooking time: 50 minutes
6 servings

Gently cook the onions and shallots in a non-stick frying pan with 6 tablespoons water. Stir from time to time, then deglaze with the white wine. Add the crème fraîche and leave to simmer for 5 minutes over a low heat. Add the scallops, prawns and mussels.

Combine all the ingredients very thoroughly and leave to simmer for a further 20 minutes. Preheat the oven to 180°C/350°F/Gas 4.

Arrange six ramekin dishes on a baking tray and divide the scallop mixture between them. Bake in the oven for 20 minutes.

60. Whelks

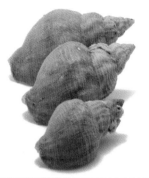

A highly prized shellfish whose increasing popularity is threatening the species' extinction, whelks have a lot of bite but are also very filling, very low in calories and easy to eat. Most important, since they have to be winkled out of their shells, whelks are another one for my 'slow foods' category, foods that automatically make fast eaters slow down the pace at which they devour their meals.

General nutritional characteristics
As regards nutrition, whelks are nothing but good news! Lean (1g fat per 100g), stuffed with proteins (19.4g per 100g), and all this for only 88 calories.

Role in the Dukan Diet
Whelks more or less have everything going for them in my diet: they are healthy as they contain iodine, high in protein, unusual and useful as an aperitif snack. Their only downside is their price, which keeps going up. So enjoy them while you can!

How to prepare and eat whelks in the Dukan Diet
You can only eat them cooked. Be careful – the bigger they are, the firmer they are too. There are many different ways of cooking them. Put some whelks in a litre (1¾ pints) of cold water with 30g (1oz) sea salt, a bouquet garni and some pepper. Let them boil for 20 minutes then serve with Dukan mayonnaise (see page 222) or aïoli (garlic mayonnaise). They are also delicious grilled and served with a curry sauce.

Whelks sautéed with garlic and parsley

Bulots sautés à l'ail doux et persil plat

Salt and black pepper
100ml (3½fl oz) white wine
  vinegar
1 onion
1 carrot, sliced
1 bouquet garni
1 garlic bulb plus 4 extra
  cloves
4 bay leaves

1.6kg (3lb 8oz) shelled whelks
8 sprigs fresh flat-leaf parsley,
  chopped

Phase 1 PP / Phase 2 PP

Preparation time: 10 minutes
Cooking time: 30 minutes
4 servings

Bring a large pan of water to the boil and add some salt and black pepper. Add the vinegar, onion, carrot, bouquet garni, garlic bulb and bay leaves and bring back to the boil. Once the water is boiling, add the whelks and cook for 30 minutes over a medium heat. When the whelks are cooked, remove them from the water and leave them to cool.

Cut the whelks into small pieces then gently fry them in a little water in a non-stick frying pan along with the extra garlic cloves and parsley. If necessary, adjust the seasoning.

Arrange the whelks on a plate, piling them up high, and serve them immediately, piping hot.

61. Hen's eggs

Found and enjoyed in every culture, eggs are almost a complete food in themselves. They are easy to cook with and very filling despite their low calorie content.

General nutritional characteristics

One egg contains about 80 calories, of which 68 are found in the yolk and 12 in the egg white; 6.5g of proteins, half in the yolk and half in the white; no carbohydrate or fibre but a lot of iron and vitamins A and E – two of the best anti-oxidants – vitamin D and a wide range of B vitamins.

Role in the Dukan Diet

Eggs are a foundation food in my diet for several reasons. They are up there with the most filling foods in the world alongside tinned tuna in brine, chicken liver and prawns. So, if you have been invited out for a long supper where your dieting may be put at risk, do not think twice about grabbing a hard-boiled egg half an hour beforehand. Eggs contain 270mg of cholesterol, which is the only factor limiting their use, but this should concern only those with high cholesterol. At worst, four eggs a week should worry nobody, especially when following a diet that has no other added fats.

How to prepare and eat hen's eggs in the Dukan Diet

Eggs can be prepared in so many different ways. Soft- and hard-boiled, fried or in an omelette, coddled or scrambled. You should be aware that how quickly an egg is digested, and therefore how much it will fill you up, depends on how it is cooked: two soft-boiled eggs pass through the stomach in 105 minutes; raw eggs take longer, 135 minutes, while fried eggs take 151 minutes and hard-boiled eggs 170 minutes. Of course, eggs are an ingredient in custards, soufflés, the famous oat bran galette and all sorts of mixed salads such as the French classic *salade niçoise*.

Mexican-style poached eggs
Œufs pochés à la mexicaine

1 white onion, thinly sliced
1 green pepper, deseeded and
  diced
½ teaspoon chilli powder
1 garlic clove, crushed
2 tomatoes, skinned and diced
800g (1lb 12oz) tomato
  passata
Salt and black pepper
4 eggs

Phase 2 PV

Preparation time: 10 minutes
Cooking time: 20 minutes
4 servings

Gently fry the onion and pepper for 10 minutes with 4 tablespoons water. Add the chilli powder, garlic, tomatoes, passata and one glass of water. Bring the mixture to the boil, lower the heat and leave to simmer, covered, for 10 minutes. Season with salt and black pepper.

In the meantime, prepare the poached eggs. Put a pan of water on to boil. Break each egg into a small cup. Once the water is boiling, bring a cup to the surface of the water and, in a single movement; flip the cup over. Continue with the other eggs, positioning them in different areas of the pan.

After 3 minutes, remove the eggs using a draining spoon and arrange them on top of the vegetables.

62. Quail's eggs

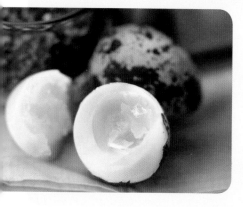

Apart from being smaller, which means they appeal to children and make a change from eating hen's eggs, quail's eggs are also of nutritional interest since they have anti-allergy properties.

General nutritional characteristics

A quail's egg yolk is, proportionately, 30% bigger than a hen's egg yolk, which means it also has a proportionately higher cholesterol content. However, of particular interest to women is that quail's eggs are seven times richer in iron and 15 times richer in vitamin B12, and both can help those who suffer from heavy periods and who are prone to anaemia. Lastly, quail's eggs are high in arachidonic acid, a fatty acid with good anti-allergy properties.

Role in the Dukan Diet

In my diet, quail's eggs are particularly useful for those occasions when you are most at risk: for example, when there are aperitif snacks on offer. Quail's eggs team up well with cherry tomatoes to provide a tasty alternative, so you can avoid succumbing to the worst of temptations – crisps and peanuts. Furthermore, quail's eggs are very satisfying and take some time to shell. At the end of the day, or whenever you feel a little peckish, they can help keep hunger pangs at bay.

How to prepare and eat quail's eggs in the Dukan Diet

Quail's eggs are prepared in just the same way as hen's eggs. They are mainly eaten hard-boiled and are easy to carry around and consume when you're out and about, a little like protein 'sweets'. Dishes such as jellied quail's eggs, poached quail's eggs on top of artichoke hearts or scrambled quail's eggs with truffle shavings show that there are no limits to what a creative imagination can conjure up.

Quail's eggs wrapped in bacon
Œufs de caille au bacon

20 quail's eggs
10 thin slices fat-reduced
  bacon

Phase 1 PP / Phase 2 PP

Preparation time: 15 minutes
Cooking time: 10 minutes
2 servings

Boil the quail's eggs in water until they are hard, about 7 minutes.

Meanwhile, cut the bacon slices in half and fry them in a non-stick frying pan.

Shell the quail's eggs and wrap the bacon slices around them, using wooden cocktail sticks to keep them in place. Serve hot.

63. Cottage cheese (low fat)

In most English-speaking countries, low-fat cottage cheese makes a fantastic contribution to the Dukan Diet; unfortunately it is not available in France – but the French could really use it! Cottage cheese has a slightly sour taste, and chewy, chunky texture, and it is very filling.

General nutritional characteristics

As far as nutrition is concerned, cottage cheese is a fantastic source of calcium and proteins of excellent quality, which is very beneficial for women over 40. As it contains hardly any lactose at all, you can eat it without restriction.

Role in the Dukan Diet

Cottage cheese is extremely useful in my diet as it can be carried around so easily, it keeps for ages and it fills you up quickly.

How to prepare and eat cottage cheese in the Dukan Diet

More often than not, cottage cheese is eaten straight from the pot by the spoonful, as it is one of the most popular dairy products for people following the diet. It can be used in a great many recipes. For example, you can make a Greek-style tzatziki or season and flavour some cottage cheese to be used as stuffing for quails. For those of you who have little time for lunch, the best recipe is an oat bran galette covered generously with cottage cheese, topped with a nice slice of smoked salmon and then garnished with a little dill and lemon.

Cottage cheese and salmon roe roulade

Roulés aux œufs de saumon et au cottage cheese

6 eggs, separated
500g (1lb 2oz) virtually fat-free
  cottage cheese
Handful of chopped
  fresh chives
Salt and black pepper
2 gelatine leaves
6 tablespoons 3% fat crème
  fraîche

4 slices smoked salmon
1 small jar salmon roe

Phase 1 PP / 2 PP

Preparation time: 35 minutes
Cooking time: 15 minutes +
  overnight chilling
6 servings

Preheat the oven to 180°C/350°F/Gas 4 and line an ovenproof dish with greaseproof paper.

Beat the egg yolks into 125g (4½oz) of the cottage cheese and add some of the chives. Season with salt and black pepper.

Whisk the egg whites until stiff and then gently fold them into the egg yolk mixture. Spread this 'pastry' mixture over the greaseproof paper and bake in the oven for 12 minutes.

Soak the gelatine in some cold water for 5 minutes then drain and mix into the remaining cottage cheese with the crème frâiche and the remaining chives. Season with salt and black pepper.

Once the pastry is cooked, spread the cottage cheese mixture over it, add the smoked salmon slices and scatter the salmon roe on top, then roll up the pastry to make a roulade. Wrap the roulade in clingfilm and leave in the fridge overnight.

The following day, remove the clingfilm and cut the roulade into slices.

64. Fat-free fromage frais

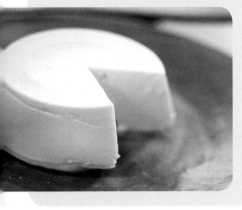

If we had to compare yoghurt with fromage frais, leaving aside our own personal taste preferences, fromage frais would win by a short head and for two very simple reasons. First, fromage frais is more compact and therefore slightly more satisfying and, second, it contains more proteins and is a little less acidic. Yoghurt is nonetheless more widely used than fromage frais, probably because it comes in many more different varieties.

General nutritional characteristics

Fromage frais has the same nutritional qualities as yoghurt and, as with yoghurt, you can eat as much as you want of the natural or flavoured fat-free types. However, you are not allowed any fromage frais with fruit. As far as nutrition goes, non-fat fromage frais is an obvious source of protein with a high nutritional value. It contains very little lactose but lots of calcium. You get bags of flavour and it fills you up into the bargain!

Role in the Dukan Diet

Fat-free fromage frais, like all non-fat dairy products, plays a crucial role in my diet. There are several brands of fat-free fromage frais, every supermarket chain has its own version and there is not a lot to choose between them – they all promise 'a real treat' for only 60 calories per 100g.

How to prepare and eat fromage frais in the Dukan Diet

Fat-free fromage frais can be eaten as it is or with sweetener, and as an ingredient in a whole range of different dishes.

Fluffy strawberry mousse
Mousse aérienne à la fraise

3 gelatine leaves
2–3 tablespoons sweetener
2 teaspoons strawberry
  flavouring (www.
  mydukandietshop.co.uk)
5 drops red food colouring
  (optional)
4 egg whites
Pinch of salt

400g (14oz) fat-free fromage
  frais

Phase 1 PP / Phase 2 PP

Preparation time: 20 minutes
Cooking time: 10–15 minutes
  (for the syrup) + 4 hours chilling
4 servings

Soak the gelatine leaves in cold water for 5 minutes, then drain.

Bring the sweetener and 4 tablespoons water to the boil in a pan and simmer for 2 minutes. Add the strawberry flavouring, drained gelatine leaves and food colouring (if using). Stir and remove from the heat.

In a large bowl, whisk the egg whites with the salt until stiff – the salt makes them stiffer. Drizzle in the syrup very gradually, whisking all the time. Next fold in the fromage frais very gently so that you do not break up the egg whites.

Divide the mixture equally between four dessert dishes and refrigerate for 4 hours.

65. Fat-free Greek yoghurt

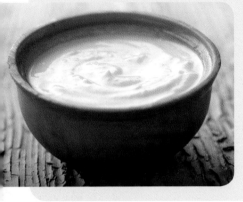

Along with Bulgarian yoghurt, Greek yoghurt is one of the best known in the world. Generally it is produced from whole milk, and cream may even be added to make it richer. However, the fat-free version from which the lipids have been removed still manages to preserve a distinctive and sufficiently pleasant taste for you to forget that there is no fat.

General nutritional characteristics

As far as nutrition goes, fat-free Greek yoghurt is brimming with good-quality proteins; and, like all reduced-fat dairy products, it is high in calcium and low in lactose. Full of lactobacilli, yoghurt enables intestinal flora to replenish, which can be advantageous if you suffer from flatulence. Current research on the role that intestinal flora play in the process of putting on weight might explain yoghurt's part (especially that of Greek yoghurt) in helping people to lose weight.

Role in the Dukan Diet

In my diet, fat-free Greek yoghurt is an extremely useful ingredient as it is easily found in supermarkets. It gives the diet an almost therapeutic taste and quality since Greece is the country of origin of the Cretan diet, famous for being healthy.

How to prepare and eat fat-free Greek yoghurt in the Dukan Diet

Fat-free Greek yoghurt comes into its own when used in tzatziki, the Greek starter, or mezze, that is extremely popular all over the world and is made by mixing grated cucumber, crushed garlic, finely chopped mint and coriander, salt and pepper into the yoghurt

Seafood stick salad with Greek yoghurt

Salade de surimi au yaourt à la grecque

1 cucumber
600g (1lb 5oz) seafood sticks, grated
4 tomatoes
450g (1lb) fat-free Greek yoghurt
Handful of chopped fresh chives

Juice of 1 lemon
Salt and black pepper

Phase 2 PV

Preparation time: 20 minutes + 30 minutes resting
4 servings

Dice the cucumber and leave for 30 minutes to allow any water to drain off.

Chop the tomatoes into small cubes. Mix together the Greek yoghurt, chives and lemon juice and season with salt and black pepper.

Stir the tomatoes, cucumber and grated seafood sticks into the Greek yoghurt sauce and serve well chilled.

66. Fat-free yoghurt

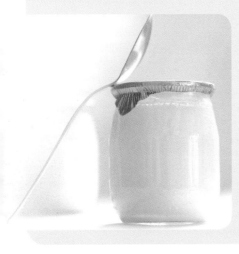

Along with aspartame, diet fizzy drinks, sugar-free chewing gum, oat bran, balsamic vinegar, low-fat sliced meats and seafood sticks, fat-free yoghurt is the product that provides the most help for people struggling with weight problems. To their credit these items have probably helped dieters all over the world to control their weight; they have eased pathologies and made months if not years of human lives easier. This means that yoghurt is a fundamental element in the diet.

General nutritional characteristics

Like all dairy products, yoghurt contains lactose which provides slower-release sugars and alleviates ketosis if you are dieting with artificial protein sachets. There are 40–50 calories per small pot.

Role in the Dukan Diet

For my diet, fat-free yoghurt is a real godsend. By definition it contains no fat and no added sugar. The yoghurt can be flavoured and is satisfyingly creamy, refreshing, easy to carry around in pots, full of calcium and very high-quality proteins but low in calories. In the Dukan Diet a yoghurt is the simplest and most natural way to finish off a meal.

How to prepare and eat yoghurt in the Dukan Diet

There are three types of fat-free yoghurt. Natural yoghurt is smooth and velvety, with a thickish or fluid texture; you can eat as much as you want of it. Flavoured yoghurt – vanilla, coconut, lemon, lychee, etc. – you can also eat as much as you like. And then there are fruit yoghurts – such a myriad out there that it would take an army of experts a year to test them all! For fruit yoghurts the instruction is simple: they are banned. If you are absolutely desperate you can have one as a back-up, but only if your personal coach gives permission.

Yoghurt cake
Gâteau au yaourt

150g (5½oz) fat-free yoghurt
4 eggs
4 tablespoons oat bran
2 tablespoons wheat bran
6 tablespoons powdered
  skimmed milk
1 teaspoon baking powder
1 teaspoon liquid sweetener, or
  more according to taste

Flavouring of your choice
(www.mydukandietshop.co.uk)

Phase 1 PP / Phase 2 PP

Preparation time: 10 minutes
Cooking time: 30 minutes
2 servings

Preheat the oven to 150°C/300°F/Gas 2.

In a large bowl, mix together the yoghurt and eggs. Add the brans, powdered milk, baking powder, sweetener and a few drops of flavouring if you would like your cake to have a particular flavour.

Pour the mixture into a cake tin and bake in the oven for 30 minutes.

67. Quark (low fat)

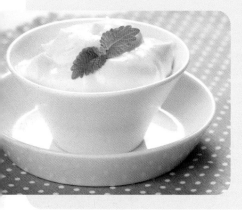

Quark is a dairy product that comes originally from Germany, where it is a real institution. It is available in all supermarkets and is similar to cream cheese, although its creaminess is slightly offset by a delicate hint of saltiness. Quark has a slightly granular texture and is thick enough to be used as a spread.

General nutritional characteristics

As far as nutrition goes, virtually fat-free quark contains a lot of protein and calcium but very little carbohydrate. It has around 67–73 calories per 100g.

Role in the Dukan Diet

Filling, virtually fat-free, packed with high-quality vitamins, like all non-fat dairy products quark plays a key role in my diet and method.

How to prepare and eat quark in the Dukan Diet

Quark can be used as a spread on oat bran galettes. It is particularly delicious when mixed with finely chopped herbs and it can be substituted for mozzarella to make a lovely starter with tomatoes. Equally, quark can be transformed into a pudding by sprinkling over some sweetener, the faint hint of saltiness producing an unusual taste combination. Quark can be used extensively in cooking and baking.

Dukan taramasalata

Tarama Dukan

100g (3½oz) salmon, red
  lumpfish or cod roe
70g (2½oz) virtually fat-free
  quark
15g (½oz) fat-free fromage
  frais
Juice of ½ lemon
½ teaspoon mild paprika

1 egg white, stiffly beaten
  (optional)

Phase 1 PP / Phase 2 PP

**Preparation time: 10 minutes +
  1 hour chilling
1 serving**

Using a fork, crush the roe in a large bowl. Add the quark, fromage frais, lemon juice and paprika. If you would prefer a lighter mixture, you can also add 1 stiffly beaten egg white.

Refrigerate for at least 1 hour. Spread the mixture generously over a Dukan galette (see page 161).

68. Skimmed milk

Since it arrived on the scene, skimmed milk – once used only for people suffering from liver complaints – has become one of the key foods in weight-loss diets, and most especially in mine. This is why it has a very important place among my 100 foods.

General nutritional characteristics

Milk contains a lot of proteins with a high nutritional value; some carbohydrates, including, of course, lactose; and lots of calcium. For those who can use it in the right quantities, powdered skimmed milk has many advantages. It keeps for a long time and does not go off like fresh milk in a carton. It is cheaper and you can make it more or less concentrated, depending on your taste, appetite or what you are making.

Role in the Dukan Diet

For people who like milk and are not lactose intolerant, skimmed milk is a real boon as it is both food and drink. Very cheap and extremely filling, milk gives the diet cohesion and makes it easier to follow as it is used in so many different recipes and snacks.

How to prepare and eat skimmed milk in the Dukan Diet

There are too many recipes for us to consider them all here, but one of the easiest and quickest snacks (or desserts) is a custard flan, flavoured with vanilla, coffee, cinnamon or fat-reduced cocoa. Try adding milk to pumpkin soup. And, of course, we drink milk in tea, coffee and fat-reduced cocoa. For people with a really hearty appetite and those who love to snack, milk is an ideal solution. Why not try some skimmed milk flavoured with vanilla?

Pistachio-flavoured eggs in milk
Œufs au lait arôme pistache

1 litre (1¾ pints) skimmed milk	2 drops blue food colouring (optional)	**Phase 1 PP / Phase 2 PP**
1 cardamom pod, seeds removed	2 drops yellow food colouring (optional)	**Preparation time: 5 minutes** **Cooking time: 30 minutes +** **2 hours chilling**
6 eggs		**4–8 servings**
2 tablespoons pistachio flavouring (www. mydukandietshop.co.uk)		
4 tablespoons liquid sweetener		

Preheat the oven to 150°C/300°F/Gas 2.

Put the milk and cardamom seeds in a saucepan and bring to the boil. Remove from the heat and leave to infuse for 15 minutes.

In the meantime, break the eggs into a large bowl and whisk them together using an egg whisk. Add the flavouring and the sweetener and combine thoroughly.

Add the warm milk, whisking continuously. Finish off with the drops of food colouring (if using) and whisk them in. Divide the mixture between four or eight ramekin dishes, depending on size, and place them on a baking tray. Bake in the oven for 30 minutes.

Remove the ramekins from the oven, leave to cool to room temperature, then refrigerate for 2 hours.

69. Konjac

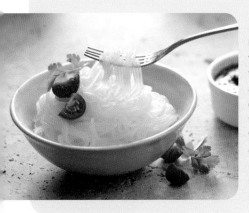

Konjac is a plant root, like an enormous beetroot, which has been eaten in Japan for centuries. For anyone wanting to lose weight, Konjac Shirataki noodles are an absolute godsend. The Japanese cook extensively with Konjac and Japanese women along with French women share the prize for being the slimmest women on earth with the longest life span. Konjac can be used in many different recipes and deserves to be more widely known.

General nutritional characteristics

It is the glucomannan, the fibre in Konjac, that makes it so special (2.2g per 100g); and, like pectin in apples and beta-glucans in oat bran, it has a great future ahead. This fibre can absorb up to 100 times its weight in water, forming an extremely viscous gel that fills the stomach while trapping fats and sugars. What is magical is that there are almost *no calories* (9 per 100g), yet Konjac is really filling, which is why I became interested early on in this amazing miracle food.

Role in the Dukan Diet

Konjac comes in different forms (blocks, vermicelli, powder, etc.), but to my mind the best way to eat it is as noodles, or Shirataki. Nowadays, there are vermicelli and noodle products that keep very well. The noodles look like pasta, have practically no calories and are cooked in exactly the same way as vermicelli or spaghetti. They are slightly chewy and have a very pleasant texture but no particular flavour of their own; they soak up the taste of the sauce or whatever they are mixed with.

How to prepare and eat Konjac noodles in the Dukan Diet

The standard way of serving Konjac noodles for the Dukan Diet is with a bolognaise sauce made with mince and a shop-bought or homemade tomato sauce, which must be fat- and sugar-free. You can eat Konjac noodles in the Attack phase – just cut down the tomato sauce to one tablespoon while sticking with the mince. In the Cruise phase you can add all sorts of vegetables to the noodles, such as diced aubergine and courgette, strips of pepper, etc.

Konjac Shirataki noodles with clams

Shiratakis de Konjac aux clovisses

2 packs Konjac Shirataki
  noodles (www.
  mydukandietshop.co.uk)
1 onion, chopped
2 garlic cloves, finely chopped
600g (1lb 5oz) clams, tinned
Salt and black pepper
250g (9oz) cherry tomatoes,
  halved

Handful of fresh basil, finely
  chopped

Phase 2 PV

Preparation time: 20 minutes
Cooking time: 20 minutes
4 servings

Rinse the noodles in plenty of cold water and bring a large pan of water to the boil. Add the noodles and cook for 2 minutes, then drain, rinse under some cold water and put to one side.

Add three drops of oil to a non-stick frying pan and wipe off with kitchen paper. Gently fry the onion for 5–6 minutes, then add the garlic and clams and season with salt and black pepper. Cook, stirring all the time, to heat through and then add the cherry tomatoes. Continue to cook until all the ingredients have softened down.

Once the sauce is ready, add the Konjac Shirataki noodles and basil to the frying pan and stir everything together thoroughly. Cook for a further 3 minutes before serving.

70. Oat bran

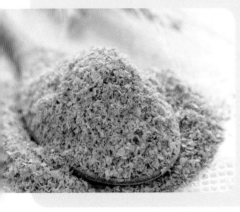

For a long time, this foodstuff was looked down upon and used only for feeding horses or stuffing mattresses. Nowadays, it is considered to be one of the most invaluable and health-giving foods we humans have!

General nutritional characteristics

Everything has been said about oat bran's nutritional qualities in the oat bran section of the introduction to this book. However, the following should be reiterated: oat bran has a high protein content; it has a great capacity to soak up liquid (up to 30 times its volume in water) and fill up your stomach; and it has been proven that it reduces cholesterol, slows down the absorption of sugars, promotes bowel regularity and helps prevent bowel cancer.

Role in the Dukan Diet

Oat bran is more than a master food; it is a key food, a strategic food that considerably widens the scope of my diet. This is all down to its beta-glucan molecules, which are so viscous and adhesive that they stick to everything around them in the fatty, sugary and extremely calorific juices in the food bolus. So with oat bran we have a new type of food, an anti-food which sneaks away the very best calories from the foods we eat.

How to prepare and eat oat bran in the Dukan Diet

Oat bran's other excellent qualities come to light in the many different ways it can be prepared: it tastes good; it is flavoursome and hugely filling, and lends itself to all sorts of surprising uses in an effective slimming diet. It all started off with the galette, then came the crêpes, the blinis, the bread, the pizza, the pancakes, the biscuits and so on. Those who are pushed for time simply add bran to their yoghurt, thereby giving it the taste, texture and crunchiness of cereals. Lots of people make porridge in the microwave with oat bran and sweetened skimmed milk.

Dukan oat bran galette

Galette aux sons Dukan

3 tablespoons oat bran
2 tablespoons fat-free fromage
  frais
1 egg

Phase 1 PP / Phase 2 PP

Preparation time: 5 minutes
Cooking time: 6 minutes
1 serving

In a large bowl, mix together all the ingredients. Oil a non-stick frying pan with a few drops of oil and wipe away with kitchen paper.

Cook the galette over a medium heat for about 3 minutes, until it comes away from the bottom of the pan, then turn it over and cook the other side.

You can make the galette with just the egg white (preferably whisked) if you have high cholesterol or wish to cut back on the number of egg yolks you eat.

For a savoury galette, add your choice of herbs and spices, or enjoy a sweet version by adding some sweetener.

71. Tofu

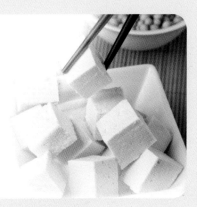

Tofu is made from soya milk curds that have been shaped and then compressed. It is a Japanese product which, like seafood sticks, has gradually become popular across the world because of its particular qualities. Sold in rectangular blocks, tofu has a texture varying between that of custard and feta cheese and it is still not that widely known or used in Western Europe.

General nutritional characteristics
Tofu's composition is very similar to that of lean meat (16g proteins, 8g fats, 1g of carbohydrates per 100g), with only 142 calories per 100g. Moreover, it contains lots of iron and magnesium and it has *absolutely no* cholesterol.

Role in the Dukan Diet
Tofu has an important place in my diet as it is one of the only plant foods sufficiently high in protein to be included in my PP list. It contains just as much protein as fish and meat, but less fat. Its proteins are slightly less complete than animal proteins; they lack one essential amino acid, methionine, so there is a 'gap' in their structure which prevents them from being absorbed. To get round this, all you need to do is combine tofu with oat bran, the only cereal allowed in my diet, because it contains so much methionine it gives these proteins the same biological value as animal proteins.

How to prepare and eat tofu in the Dukan Diet
Uncooked, tofu can be diced, seasoned and added to salads or starters. It can be fried, grilled on a griddle pan, slowly cooked or even braised. The blandness of tofu is easily livened up by adding onions and garlic, soy sauce, ginger, curry spices, Dijon or Meaux mustard, chilli powder and, of course, some Worcestershire sauce.

Silken tofu mousse
Mousse au tofu soyeux

500ml (18fl oz) skimmed milk
Juice and grated zest of 1
  lemon
½ teaspoon ground cinnamon
300g (10½oz) silken tofu
3 tablespoons powdered
  sweetener, or more
  according to taste

200g (7oz) virtually fat-free
  quark
1 × 8g sachet powdered
  gelatine
1 teaspoon orange flower
  water

Phase 1 PP / Phase 2 PP

Preparation time: 10 minutes +
  20 minutes infusing +
  3 hours chilling
6 servings

Put the milk, lemon zest and ground cinnamon in a pan and bring to the boil. Take off the heat and leave to infuse for 20 minutes.

In a blender, blend the silken tofu with the sweetener, quark, lemon juice and the warm milk. You will have a foamy mixture that already tastes quite delicious.

Dissolve the gelatine in a little water. Pour the tofu mixture into a saucepan and gently warm it so you can stir in the gelatine and whisk it all together. Then leave the mixture to cool a little before pouring it into glass dishes.

Leave the mousse to cool down to room temperature, then refrigerate for 3 hours before serving.

72. Artichoke (globe)

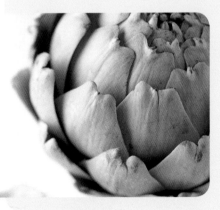

Only the fleshy part of the flower from this cultivated vegetable is edible. Globe artichokes belong to my 'slow foods' category – you have to remove all the leaves before you can start eating and this takes time! Artichokes would be one of the very best slimming foods if they did not contain quite as many calories (40 per 100g); however, this slight drawback is balanced by the satiety they offer and their texture, which is both chewy and dense.

General nutritional characteristics
Artichokes contain a moderate amount of calories: 80 in a nice 200g (7oz). Rich in potassium and phosphorus, they have a slightly diuretic detox effect; they are also choleretic (stimulating bile production in the liver) and a powerful 'cleanser' for your liver. Because of this, artichokes are a great slimming aid, especially for women who suffer with water retention and for seriously obese people with tired livers. They contain a lot of iron, magnesium and vitamins that promote tone and fight fatigue (C, B1, B12).

Role in the Dukan Diet
Artichokes are eaten leaf by leaf, so you are forced to eat slowly and this helps you to start to feel full. Of all fresh vegetables, they are also one of the richest sources of proteins, which this increases their nutritional density and their ability to make you feel replete.

How to prepare and eat artichoke in the Dukan Diet
Artichokes can be eaten hot or cold after being cooked in water or steamed (eat straightaway otherwise they will oxidize). Dip the end of the leaves into some Dukan vinaigrette dressing (see page 223) or balsamic vinegar. Once you strip the artichoke down to its centre, discard the straw-like fibres to reveal the warm, tender heart. This has an exceptional texture and mild flavour because it contains inulin, a very slow carbohydrate. Artichoke hearts can also be eaten raw – slice very thinly and marinate in lemon juice and salt. You can also buy frozen hearts, which can be used to stuff white meat or make a handy accompaniment or vegetable macedoine served with a slice of smoked salmon on top. To avoid flatulence, be careful to cook them properly.

Artichokes stuffed with prawns
Artichauts farcis aux crevettes

2 handfuls shelled, cooked
  small prawns
Juice of 2 large lemons
Salt and black pepper
2 generous tablespoons
  fat-free yoghurt
2 teaspoons mustard
2 tablespoons balsamic
  vinegar

Fresh herbs of your choice,
  chopped
4 large artichoke hearts,
  cooked

Phase 2 PV

Preparation time: 10 minutes
2 servings

Marinate the prawns in the lemon juice. Season with some salt and black pepper.

Mix together the yoghurt, mustard, balsamic vinegar and fresh herbs to make a sauce. Chop 2 of the artichoke hearts along with the prawns and stir them into the sauce. Use this mixture to spread over and fill the remaining 2 hearts and serve them cold.

73. Asparagus

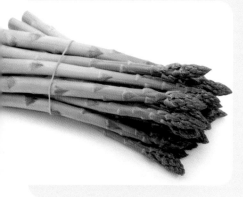

Since asparagus is not terribly filling, it is only moderately useful as a slimming vegetable. Associated with luxury and fine dining, it is expensive and not enjoyed by everyone. Asparagus is only eaten cooked, never raw.

General nutritional characteristics

Asparagus is very low in calories, with 24 per 100g. A diuretic, it is very quickly eliminated from the body with an unpleasant, strong smell which more elegant eaters may find off-putting; it may even irritate sensitive urinary tracts.

Role in the Dukan Diet

Green asparagus is good to try when in season and is rather attractive and festive. White asparagus is less stringy with a denser texture, but is very expensive, especially when tinned. However, it is very useful if your diet needs some variety.

How to prepare and eat asparagus in the Dukan Diet

When served warm, asparagus cries out for hollandaise sauce, but this is packed with calories and must be replaced by a Dukan mayonnaise (see page 222). When cold, asparagus needs only some coriander vinaigrette to intensify and strengthen the flavour, or alternatively some very thick but mild mustard sauce (the grainy Moutarde de Meaux *à l'ancienne* works well). You can also use asparagus tips in omelettes, with scrambled eggs or in mixed salads. You may be able to buy frozen asparagus from your supermarket.

Asparagus terrinee
Terrine d'asperges

500g (1lb 2oz) white
  asparagus
150g (5½oz) fat-free fromage
  frais
8 eggs
100g (3½oz) low-fat double
  cream
Salt and black pepper
1 teaspoon pink peppercorns

Phase 2 PV

Preparation time: 10 minutes
Cooking time: 40 minutes
4 servings

Preheat the oven to 180°C/350°F/Gas 4.

Trim and wash the asparagus and cook in salted, boiling water. Squeeze
the water out of the asparagus and then blend in a food processor or
liquidizer. Put the blended asparagus in a large bowl and combine with
the fromage frais, eggs, cream, salt and black pepper. Use a whisk to mix
together thoroughly.

Use some kitchen paper to oil a terrine dish lightly, then pour in the
asparagus mixture. Bake in the oven in a bain-marie for 40 minutes.
Remove from the oven and sprinkle over the pink peppercorns. Serve
warm.

74. Aubergine

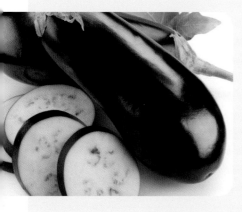

A vegetable-fruit from the Mediterranean region, the aubergine is available all year round. One of the least calorific vegetables, it stands on a par with lettuce and French beans. It is only ever eaten cooked and lends itself to many different dishes that often use far too much oil. Here lies a great danger: because of their texture, aubergines soak up oil. So avoid eating them unless you prepare them at home yourself.

General nutritional characteristics

Low in calories, aubergines contain 22 per 100g, having 4.5g carbohydrates and 91.2g water.

Role in the Dukan Diet

Aubergines play a major role in my diet because of their high pectin content. Among vegetables, they have the highest pectin content along with courgettes and pumpkin. Pectin can expand up to 30 times its weight in water, which makes it a great appetite suppressant as it fills up the stomach. Even better, once in the digestive tract pectin turns into a gel and whatever surrounds it (nutrients and calories) gets trapped in this gel's chain structure. As pectin is not absorbed by the body, it exits in the stools, taking with it a small booty of calories. Aubergines soak up any flavours in proximity – be they meat, fish, herbs or spices – and absorb them during the cooking process.

How to prepare and eat aubergine in the Dukan Diet

Aubergines can be blended to make a puréed dip, cooked in the oven, sliced and grilled, griddled, used in ratatouille, and are delicious stuffed.

Stuffed aubergines
Aubergines farcies

250g (9oz) minced beefsteak (5% fat)

250g (9oz) fat-free, rind-free pre-cooked ham slices, chopped

2 garlic cloves, chopped

150g (5½oz) mushrooms, sliced

1 onion, finely chopped

2 tablespoons tomato purée

Salt and black pepper

4 aubergines, halved and deseeded

Nutritional yeast

Phase 2 PV

Preparation time: 15 minutes
Cooking time: 30 minutes
4-6 servings

Preheat the oven to 220°C/425°F/Gas 7.

Make the stuffing by combining the minced steak, ham, garlic, mushrooms and onion. Bind the mixture with the tomato purée. Season with salt and black pepper and divide among the aubergines. Sprinkle over the nutritional yeast and bake in the oven for 30 minutes.

75. Beetroot

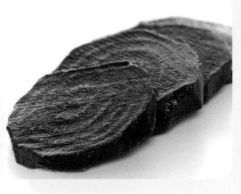

Beetroot has a low nutritional value and is a vegetable that not everyone enjoys, so why have I included it in my 100 foods? Take a look at the role it plays in my diet and you will understand!

General nutritional characteristics
Beetroot has only slightly more calories than other vegetables (40, and 8g carbohydrates per 100g). It has a very low vitamin content but lots of oxalic acid and so should be avoided if you have a history of stones in the urinary tract.

Role in the Dukan Diet
Beetroot has just one thing going for it in my diet, but it is highly significant: of all my foods it is the only one with a purely sweet taste – enough to be of use to anyone wanting a natural sugar taste rather than that of an artificial sweetener, yet this does not stop the diet from being effective as beetroot contains only 8g carbohydrates per 100g and these are slow carbohydrates. Some other vegetables have a slight sweetness, such as carrots, pumpkin and celeriac, but none of these comes close to competing with beetroot's downright sweet flavour.

How to prepare and eat beetroot in the Dukan Diet
Beetroot is eaten cooked (you can often buy it ready-cooked) and it is used in starters or colourful salads.

Beetroot mimosa

Betterave mimosa

1 cooked beetroot
2 hard-boiled eggs
Dukan vinaigrette dressing
  (see page 223)
Salt and black pepper

Phase 2 PV

Preparation time: 5 minutes
2 servings

Peel the beetroot and slice it into a dish. Remove the yolks from the hard-boiled eggs and grate them over the beetroot. Add some Dukan vinaigrette dressing, season with salt and black pepper, and serve.

76. Broccoli

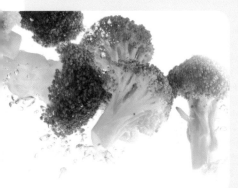

An excellent slimming food, broccoli is very filling and has an unusual flavour. When it is cooked, the stalks are crunchy and the heads have a granular texture. A relatively recent arrival in our shops, broccoli – including the purple sprouting variety – has quickly become a popular vegetable, promoted particularly by Italian and Asian cooking.

General nutritional characteristics

Broccoli contains few calories: 25 per 100g. As for nutrition, a number of studies worldwide proclaim it to be the food we should eat to prevent cancer. Alongside the tomato, it is one of the most health-giving vegetables man can consume, especially anyone who is overweight. It is particularly rich in vitamin A and C, potassium, folic acid, magnesium and iron – quite a pharmacy and cure-all in one small vegetable.

Role in the Dukan Diet

Broccoli not only tastes great, it is also filling and excellent for your health – so go ahead and eat it regularly.

How to prepare and eat broccoli in the Dukan Diet

In France, broccoli is rarely eaten raw, except when served with other crudités, such as cauliflower florets and cherry tomatoes, along with drinks before a meal. Try it in salads, sliced very thinly. When preparing broccoli, be very careful not to overcook it, so that you keep its crunchiness and firmness. Take your inspiration from Chinese, Vietnamese and Thai cooking. Broccoli is delicious baked as a gratin with some Dukan béchamel sauce (see page 222) and a discreet dusting of Parmesan on top.

Broccoli and salmon mousse duo

Duo de mousse au brocoli et au saumon

For the salmon mousse
150g (5½oz) smoked salmon
8 tablespoons fat-free fromage frais
Juice of ½ lemon
Salt and black pepper

For the broccoli mousse
½ broccoli head, cooked

50g (1¾oz) virtually fat-free quark
1 tablespoon fat-free fromage frais
Juice of ½ lemon
Salt and black pepper

To garnish
Pinch of curry powder

Phase 2 PV

Preparation time: 30 minutes + 1 hour chilling
12 servings

First prepare the salmon mousse. Blend the salmon with the fromage frais and lemon juice until you have a smooth, creamy mixture. Add a little salt and black pepper and pour into 12 glass dishes. Refrigerate while you make the broccoli mixture.

Blend the broccoli, quark, fromage frais and lemon juice. Season with salt and black pepper. Add the broccoli mousse on top of the salmon mixture. Finish off with a sprinkle of curry powder and return the dishes to the fridge for 1 hour.

Take the dishes out of the fridge 10 minutes before you are ready to serve.

77. Brussels sprouts

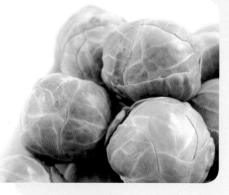

Brussels sprouts look like tiny, firm, round cabbages growing on a stick. They contain a fair few calories for a vegetable, so are not a great ally for dieters, but they are full of fibre and very filling. They can be prepared in various ways and should be kept for those people who enjoy them.

General nutritional characteristics
Like all types of cabbage, Brussels sprouts are very rich in vitamin C, folic acid and potassium and they have a reputation for protecting us against cancer. They contain 39 calories per 100g.

Role in the Dukan Diet
Unlike other types of cabbage, Brussels sprouts have to be cooked before they can be eaten.

How to prepare and eat Brussels sprouts in the Dukan Diet
Cook your sprouts in water, then you can bake them in the oven afterwards with a dusting of Parmesan on top or with some Dukan béchamel sauce (see page 222) poured over.

Puréed Brussels sprout gratin with pink trout

Gratin de purée de choux de Bruxelles à la truite rose

1kg (2lb 4oz) Brussels sprouts
4 tablespoons 3% fat crème
  fraîche
4 x 175g (6oz) salmon trout
  fillets

Phase 2 PV

Preparation time: 10 minutes
Cooking time: 20 minutes
4 servings

Preheat the oven to 180°C/350°F/Gas 4.

Cook the Brussels sprouts in a large pan of water for 5–10 minutes. When they are cooked, drain them, leave to cool and then blend them in a food processor.

Pour a layer of the puréed Brussels sprouts into each of four ramekins, then add a tablespoon of the crème fraîche, then a trout fillet. Finish off with a final layer of the Brussels sprout purée. Bake in the oven for 20 minutes.

78. Cabbage

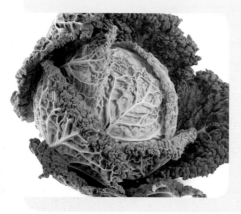

Cabbage represents a family of universal green vegetables and is one of the basic foods in mankind's gastronomic heritage. It is a great slimming food, dense and filling, but unfortunately not as attractive as, say, tomatoes or lettuce. Among all the many varieties, red cabbage stands out and entices us with its lovely colour; this is the most tender and the one that we eat most readily in salads.

General nutritional characteristics

As far as nutrition goes, cabbage, whether white or red, is the most medicinal of all vegetables and perhaps even of all foodstuffs. It is packed with health; it has the highest vitamin C content for a vegetable, and is full of folic acid, potassium and vitamin B6. It is also the food most widely acknowledged as offering protection against cancer; so families at risk should be encouraged to eat it, especially if there is any obesity too.

Role in the Dukan Diet

In my method, cabbage is a premier food, offering invaluable protection against cancer as well as a wealth of vitamins and micronutrients. Japanese catering has made cabbage fashionable with its finely chopped cabbage salads. In a restaurant just ask for it with the sauce or dressing on the side and eat only sauces that have not been sweetened. Traditionally cabbage is eaten cooked, either steamed, boiled, braised or lightly fried. It is delicious stuffed; see the recipe for stuffed cabbage opposite. You can also try eating it grated with some vinaigrette dressing.

How to prepare and eat cabbage in the Dukan Diet

Sauerkraut, if you leave aside the meat products that come with it, is a fermented vegetable dish produced by combining finely chopped cabbage with salt, which makes the cabbage more digestible. If you are careful about the meat you select to go into a sauerkraut recipe (i.e. no ham or sausages), it can be a great slimming food; any alcohol in the cooking wine evaporates but leaves behind its flavour.

Stuffed cabbage
Chou farci

1 large green cabbage
300g (10½oz) minced
beefsteak (5% fat)
1 onion, finely chopped
Salt and black pepper
2–3 tablespoons tomato
passata

Phase 2 PV

Preparation time: 10 minutes
Cooking time: 45 minutes
4 servings

Blanch the whole cabbage for a few moments in boiling water, then drain. Remove and reserve some of the outer leaves and cut out a cavity in the body of the cabbage for the stuffing.

Mix together the minced steak, onion, salt and black pepper. Fry in a non-stick frying pan and add the tomato passata. Stuff the cabbage with this mixture and use the reserved large outer leaves to close up the cabbage. Tie with a piece of cooking string.

Place the cabbage in a casserole with a little water and turn it over and over so every part gets braised. Then put a lid on the casserole and cook over a low heat for 45 minutes.

79. Carrot

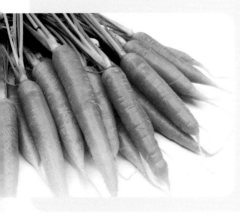

Although they contain 7g carbohydrates, twice as much as tomatoes, I still consider carrots to be an excellent slimming food. Children really enjoy them, especially when grated (this is how we often eat carrots in France) and this enjoyment continues into adulthood. The big downside of grated carrots is that they soak up too much dressing, so it is really important to add only fat-reduced versions to any grated carrot salad.

General nutritional characteristics
Carrots contain carotene, a vegetable precursor of vitamin A named after this vegetable. Carrots are one of the three major vegetables to offer us protection against a number

Role in the Dukan Diet
The slightly sweet taste of carrots, their crunchiness and the way they fill you up make for a winning combination. Do not be put off by the fact that diabetics may be apprehensive about eating carrots. Consumed raw, carrots are not absorbed by the body any more quickly than other vegetables. When carrots are eaten cooked, the sugars do enter the bloodstream more rapidly, but only diabetics need be concerned by this.

How to prepare and eat carrot in the Dukan Diet
Try eating carrots grated raw in a salad, cooked and puréed to make a mash, in soups or sliced in beef or veal stews.

Cream of carrot soup with ginger

Velouté de carottes au gingembre

4 carrots, thinly sliced
1 teaspoon ground ginger
1 low-salt chicken stock cube
1 garlic clove, chopped
1 tablespoon 3% fat single
 cream
Salt and black pepper

Phase 2 PV

Preparation time: 10 minutes
Cooking time: 10–15 minutes
2 servings

Put the carrots, ground ginger, crumbled stock cube, garlic and 500ml (18fl oz) water in a pan. Cover and cook the carrots over a gentle heat until they are tender (check with a knife – it should sink in easily). Season with a little salt and black pepper.

Blend the soup and if it is too thick add some extra water. Pour in the cream and whizz in the blender again. Adjust the seasoning as required and serve hot.

80. Cauliflower

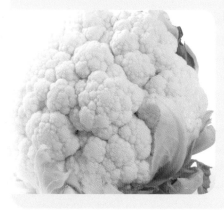

Found in all cultures, cauliflower is a universal food with a strong 'personality'. Always bear in mind that the longer a food has been in contact with mankind, the more essential it becomes to us and the more it protects us and helps keep us healthy.

General nutritional characteristics
As far as nutrition goes, cauliflower is very low in calories (24 per 100g), with 2g proteins and 5g carbohydrates per 100g, which gives the vegetable its mild flavour. Most important, it is one of the vegetables with the highest vitamin C content, which means it is a fortifying and stimulating food during the diet. Rich in potassium, it has a welcome diuretic effect for women who suffer from water retention. Also important for women, cauliflower is rich in folic acid and in vitamin B6, useful for those taking oral contraception. However, most noteworthy is that, along with broccoli, cauliflower is one of the foods offering us the greatest protection against cancer.

Role in the Dukan Diet
In my diet, cauliflower is a master food because it is substantial and filling; it can be presented and prepared in so many different ways; and it is a cheap, healthy and even medicinal food.

How to prepare and eat cauliflower in the Dukan Diet
Cauliflower can be eaten raw and used as an ingredient in salads. With aperitifs, cauliflower florets can be served as an appetizer alongside a fat-free dip. Cooked, cauliflower appears in many different guises and in a vast range of recipes, testifying to its long relationship with man. Cauliflower cheese made with a Dukan béchamel sauce (see page 222) and baked in the oven is delicious, as is cauliflower mashed with a few knobs of fat-reduced butter. Try using cauliflower as an extra ingredient in stuffing, or add it to vinegar to make a pickle.

Cumin-flavoured creamed cauliflower

Crème de chou-fleur au cumin

200g (7oz) cauliflower,
  steamed
500ml (18fl oz) skimmed milk
1 teaspoon agar-agar
1 teaspoon ground cumin
Sea salt
Szechuan pepper
70g (2½oz) sliced
  mushrooms, steamed

Phase 2 PV

Preparation time: 10 minutes
Cooking time: 45 minutes +
  4 hours chilling
4 servings

Blend the cauliflower with all the other ingredients except the mushrooms. Place the mixture in a pan, bring to the boil, then leave to simmer for 30 minutes.

Pour the mixture into four dishes and sprinkle over the mushrooms. Leave to cool to room temperature, then refrigerate for at least 4 hours.

81. Celery/celeriac

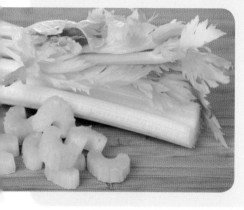

Celery is a good slimming vegetable since it is crisp and tender, the more so the closer you get to the heart. Extremely low in calories, with a strong taste and smell, celery makes a good accompaniment to many dishes. You should also try celeriac, which makes a very tasty mash.

General nutritional characteristics
Celery has very few calories indeed (15 per 100g), and is high in potassium, vitamin C and folic acid.

Role in the Dukan Diet
Celery makes a good starter when eaten raw and it teams up well with seafood, prawns and Dublin Bay prawns. When cooked, it flavours everything it comes into contact with – for example, soups, sauces for fish and poultry, as well as stews.

How to prepare and eat celery and celeriac in the Dukan Diet
Use celery with tofu, as it gives flavour to this bland protein plant food. Sliced very finely, celery changes the texture of an omelette while giving it flavour too. Braised, baked in the oven with a dusting of Parmesan on top, mixed with some oat bran or into a Dukan béchamel sauce (see page 222), celery makes a really good accompaniment. Do not throw away the leaves; wash them carefully, chop them up and add them to any food you are cooking as they will give it flavour. Celeriac is excellent as a purée served with meat or poultry and makes a great substitute for mashed potato. Celeriac can also be cut into chunks and cooked in a casserole with pieces of carrot, artichoke hearts and some lemon juice. Delicious!

Monkfish with celery hearts
Lotte aux coeurs de céleri

300g (10½oz) monkfish, cut into chunks
2 onions, finely chopped
1 low-salt fish stock cube, dissolved in 200ml (7fl oz) water
2 tinned celery hearts, halved
4 pinches of curry powder
4 tablespoons white wine
Salt and black pepper

Phase 2 PV

Preparation time: 5 minutes
Cooking time: 10 minutes
2 servings

Gently fry the monkfish in a non-stick frying pan on a bed of finely chopped onions. Pour in the fish stock. Add the celery hearts and stir well.

Cook, uncovered, for 10 minutes. Add the curry powder and white wine, and season with salt and black pepper. Serve piping hot.

82. Chicory

Witloof chicory is also called French or Belgian endive. A modern vegetable, easy to use, it keeps for a long time, is extremely low in calories, crunchy and soaks up any surrounding flavours. Its only downside is the bitter-tasting part found in the base, but if children find this bit off-putting all you need do is remove it.

General nutritional characteristics
Very low in calories (15 per 100g), chicory is the vegetable that has the most folic acid – highly recommended if you are pregnant or suffer from a cardiovascular disease – calcium and potassium. It that is slightly diuretic.

Role in the Dukan Diet
Chicory is a very good vegetable for my diet. Eaten raw, it is delicious in salads. You can either add individual leaves or cut the chicory into quarters and dress it with some Dukan vinaigrette made with balsamic vinegar (see page 223). Alternatively try it cooked with a white cheese sauce to which you can add a little blue cheese such as Roquefort or even Roquefort flavouring. As a cooked vegetable, it is mostly braised, and here it develops a distinctive, sophisticated and delicate flavour.

How to prepare and eat chicory in the Dukan Diet
Chicory can be simply braised but it will need some Dukan béchamel sauce (see page 222). The most traditional way of serving it is braised, wrapped in a slice of low-fat ham, covered with Dukan béchamel sauce and baked in the oven; and then, depending on which stage of the diet you are in and the results you have notched up, you may sprinkle over a dusting of Parmesan cheese.

Norwegian-style chicory
Endives à la norvégienne

5 chicory heads
3 slices smoked salmon
Juice of 1 lime
1 tablespoon mustard
Salt and black pepper
2 tablespoons olive oil
1 teaspoon olive flavouring
  (www.mydukandietshop.
  co.uk)
1 hard-boiled egg, chopped
	2 tablespoons chopped fresh
	  dill
	1 tablespoon pink peppercorns
		Phase 2 PV
		
		Preparation time: 10 minutes
		4 servings

Remove the outer leaves from the chicory heads, cut out the cone from the base of each and then wash and dry them. Chop the smoked salmon and slice the chicory into thin strips lengthways. Pour over 1 tablespoon of the lime juice.

In a bowl, combine the remaining lime juice with the mustard, salt and pepper. Then add the oil, olive flavouring and hard-boiled egg.

Divide the strips of chicory and chopped smoked salmon between four plates. Pour the sauce over and finish off by scattering the dill and pink peppercorns on top.

83. Courgette

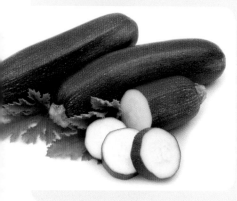

If left to mature, courgettes would turn into large marrows, but when eaten while still small they have a soft texture and are high in pectin.

General nutritional characteristics
Courgettes have only 17 calories per 100g; along with cucumbers, tomatoes, chicory and aubergines, they are one of the least calorific vegetables. Containing very little sodium but rich in potassium, they are slightly diuretic and actively help women fight water retention.

Role in the Dukan Diet
In my diet, courgettes are an absolutely necessary and useful vegetable, being very low in calories, slightly sweet-tasting and a comfort food that is extremely easy to digest. But what makes them so useful is their high pectin content, pectin being a medicinal substance capable of reducing cholesterol and the speed at which sugar is absorbed. Most important – and apple lovers will know this – pectin makes you feel full and satisfied.

How to prepare and eat courgette in the Dukan Diet
Courgettes are usually eaten cooked, either boiled or steamed, with a diet vinaigrette dressing or yoghurt sauce added. Courgettes are a ratatouille ingredient along with the three other usual suspects: tomatoes, aubergines and peppers. They make a lovely thick, creamy soup too and are good for replacing potatoes; all you need is a little low-fat cream (3% or 4% fat). You can also fry them with onions (using three drops of oil wiped off the pan with kitchen paper) and add some minced meat. Recently, using a griddle has provided another way of cooking courgettes: grilled, *al dente* and crunchy.

Cream of courgette soup
Crème de courgettes

1kg (2lb 4oz) courgettes	30g (1oz) virtually fat-free	**Phase 2 PV**
1 onion, finely chopped	quark	
1 litre (1¾ pints) fat-free	Pinch of nutmeg	**Preparation time: 15 minutes**
chicken stock	Salt and black pepper	**Cooking time: 40 minutes**
200ml (7fl oz) low fat double		**6 servings**
cream		
30g (1oz) fat-free fromage		
frais		

Peel the courgettes and cut into them into slices. Over a medium heat, warm 6 tablespoons water in a non-stick frying pan and gently fry the onion, stirring regularly, for 2 minutes. Then add the courgettes.

Pour in the chicken stock and bring everything to the boil. Cover and leave to simmer over a low heat until the courgettes are very tender (about 30 minutes). Check with the tip of a knife that the courgettes are cooked, then remove from the heat and blend the vegetables until you have a smooth mixture.

In a large bowl, combine the cream, fromage frais and quark and add to the puréed courgettes. Stir in thoroughly. Season with the nutmeg and some salt and black pepper.

If necessary, heat the soup through again in a pan before serving.

84. Cucumber

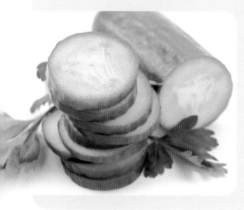

Cucumber is a food that symbolizes slimming as it contains the fewest calories of all green vegetables and it also has the least sugar and carbohydrate.

General nutritional characteristics
As far as nutrition is concerned – wait for it – cucumber has only 10 calories and 1.8g carbohydrates per 100g, yet it still provides potassium, magnesium and 1g of fibre. What a champion it is!

Role in the Dukan Diet
I give cucumber an honoured position in my diet, because as well as providing very little energy, it is rich in high-quality mineral salts such as potassium, which means it has beneficial diuretic properties. Full of water and refreshing, it is nice and crunchy and a great favourite with dieters. Lastly, it goes really well with non-fat yoghurt, which is the top slimming food in its own category.

How to prepare and eat cucumber in the Dukan Diet
Cucumber can be served in different ways: as a salad on its own or in various mixed salads, as tzatziki with yoghurt, as sticks with lemon juice; and it is also an ingredient in gazpacho.

Cucumber and quark mousse
Mousse de concombre

1 cucumber, peeled and
  deseeded
1 × 2g sachet agar-agar
200g (7oz) virtually fat-free
  quark
1 teaspoon goat's cheese
  flavouring (www.
  mydukandietshop.co.uk)
Salt and black pepper

A little chopped fresh dill
Pinch of chilli powder
  (preferably Espelette)
Radish and/or cucumber
  slices, to garnish

Phase 2 PV

Preparation time: 10 minutes
Cooking time: 5 minutes +
  1 hour chilling
2 servings

Blend the cucumber with 200ml (7fl oz) water. In a pan, dissolve the agar-agar in the cucumber mixture and bring to the boil. Simmer for 30 seconds.

Using a fork, mash the quark, and stir in the goat's cheese flavouring, a little salt, black pepper, dill and chilli powder. Stir the hot cucumber juice into the quark and pour the mixture into glass dishes. Leave to cool then refrigerate for at least 1 hour. To serve, garnish with thin slices of radish and/or cucumber.

85. Fennel

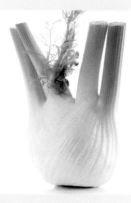

Fennel is an extremely useful slimming food as it is crunchy, fresh, filling and slightly sweet with a delicious aniseed (liquorice) flavour. It can be prepared in so many different ways and, what is more, it can be eaten both cooked and raw.

General nutritional characteristics

Containing few calories (20 per 100g), this vegetable helps with the digestion of rich dishes that are difficult to digest. Very rich in potassium, fennel contains a good amount of vitamin C and folic acid too.

Role in the Dukan Diet

What fennel offers in my diet is crunchiness, which may otherwise be missing for the many people who really enjoy eating crunchy foods. If this is the texture you are looking for, eat it raw as the Italians do, in salads with vinaigrette dressing or lemon juice. Fennel can be used as an ingredient in all types of salads where it adds a delicious aniseed fragrance and firm, crunchy freshness. Cooked, or even better lightly blanched so as not to spoil its aniseed flavour, fennel can also be braised or lightly fried as a vegetable accompaniment and can be served either on its own or with other vegetables.

How to prepare and eat fennel in the Dukan Diet

Fennel can be baked in the oven with some very low-fat cream or even grilled on a griddle pan as they do in Spain, using three drops of olive oil wiped off with kitchen paper to grease the pan. It is a good accompaniment for white meat, especially rabbit, but traditionally it is served with sea bass, a speciality that originates in Provence.

Summer seafood salad with fennel

Salade fraîcheur de la mer au fenouil

¼ medium cucumber
¼ Chinese cabbage
1 medium fennel bulb
200g (7oz) cooked prawns, shelled and cut into small pieces
300g (10½oz) seafood sticks, finely chopped
Dukan mayonnaise (see page 222)

Phase 2 PV

Preparation time: 10 minutes + 30 minutes chilling
4 servings

Peel the cucumber, then finely chop it along with the Chinese cabbage and fennel. Place the chopped vegetables in a colander and rinse under cold running water to wash them thoroughly; leave to drain in the colander.

In a large bowl, combine the vegetables with the prawns and seafood sticks and mix everything together with the Dukan mayonnaise. Place the salad in the fridge for at least 30 minutes before serving.

86. French beans

French beans are strongly associated with slimming; in fact, they are such a potent symbol that Dior dedicated a collection to lean and lanky women called the French Bean line, *la ligne Haricot Vert.*

General nutritional characteristics

French beans are an absolute nutrition bomb. Very low in calories (30 raw, 23 cooked per 100g), ultra-lean (0.2g fat per 100g) with 4g carbohydrates, they contain a lot of vitamin A – 200g (7oz) of French beans provide half a person's daily requirement. They are also rich in vitamin B1 and folic acid, essential for pregnant women.

Role in the Dukan Diet

French beans are one of the most useful vegetables in my diet – they appear in my top three. First, they contain very few calories and are one of the green vegetables with the most vegetable proteins. French beans are rich in methionine but have no lysine, which makes them an ideal partner for cereals, which conversely are rich in lysine but have little methionine. Therefore, oat bran and French beans together can create complete basic proteins for vegetarians who eat no animal meat. French beans are rich in pectin, the soluble fibre that remains for a long time in the stomach, and is extremely filling: 225g (8oz) of French beans can therefore satisfy a very strong appetite. Moreover, French beans are statistically the most popular vegetable with all groups of people, including children who are rarely tempted by vegetables. The vegetable dish most widely sold in French restaurants is French beans.

How to prepare and eat French beans in the Dukan Diet

French beans can be eaten on their own in a little vinaigrette dressing or in a mixed salad. They are mostly used as a vegetable accompaniment for meat or poultry.

French beans with bolognaise sauce

Haricots verts à la bolognaise

300–400g (10½–14oz) frozen
  French beans
1 onion, chopped
250g (9oz) minced beefsteak
  (5% fat)
Salt and black pepper
Herbes de Provence
400g (7oz) tomato passata

Phase 2 PV

Preparation time: 10 minutes
Cooking time: 35 minutes
2 servings

Cook the French beans in boiling water, then drain and put to one side to keep warm.

In a pan, gently fry the onion with 3 tablespoons water. Add the minced beef and season with salt, black pepper and herbes de Provence. Pour in the passata and leave to simmer for 30 minutes until the meat is cooked. Pour the bolognaise sauce over the French beans and serve.

87. Kohlrabi

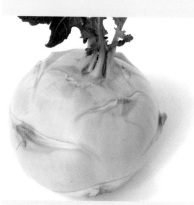

Somewhere between a cabbage and a turnip, kohlrabi will not be your greatest friend when you are slimming as it lacks colour and its texture is firm and very chewy. That said, kohlrabi does have its fans.

General nutritional characteristics

Low in calories (27 per 100g), kohlrabi contains a good amount of vitamin C and potassium. Because of its 'cabbage' origins it also helps protect against cancer.

Role in the Dukan Diet

Kohlrabi's principal contribution to my diet is the way that it can fill you up and make you feel satisfied, especially when eaten with some oil-free Dukan mayonnaise (see page 222). It also contains lots of vitamins and micronutrients. Kohlrabi can accompany poultry or it can be made into mash. Some people like to eat it steamed with the cooking juices poured over.

How to prepare and eat kohlrabi in the Dukan Diet

Kohlrabi suddenly becomes much more popular when served topped with a very low-fat cream sauce flavoured with garlic and ginger.

Kohlrabi gratin
Gratin de chou-rave

4 kohlrabis
500ml (18fl oz) skimmed milk
Salt and black pepper
2 tablespoons cornflour
Pinch of grated nutmeg

Phase 2 PV

Preparation time: 20 minutes
Cooking time: 35–45 minutes
4 servings

Peel the kohlrabis; cut them in two and then into half slices. Heat the milk in a pan and add the slices of kohlrabi and a little salt and bring to the boil. Leave to simmer very gently, uncovered, until the kohlrabi softens: between 10 and 20 minutes depending on the thickness of the slices.

Preheat the oven to 180°C/350°F/Gas 4.

Once the kohlrabi is cooked, transfer it to a gratin dish and retain the milk to make a thick Dukan béchamel sauce. Allow the milk to cool, then mix it with the cornflour. Cook for a few minutes over a low heat, stirring all the time until the sauce thickens, and season with some black pepper and a pinch of nutmeg.

Pour the sauce over the kohlrabi and bake in the oven for 35–45 minutes.

88. Lamb's lettuce

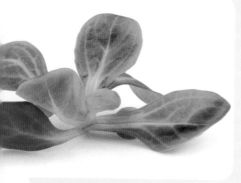

Also known as corn salad, lamb's lettuce is absolutely invaluable as a salad ingredient because of its flavour, its texture and the omega 3 fatty acids and carotene it contains.

General nutritional characteristics

As far as nutrition goes, what is of particular interest to us is just how much omega 3 fatty acids lamb's lettuce contains (half of its fats, i.e. 240mg per 100g), which has earned it the epithet of 'anti-stress salad'. It is very low in calories (12 per 100g) but very high in beta-carotene as well as vitamin E (50mg), which further increases its medicinal value.

Role in the Dukan Diet

In my diet, it ties with chicory for first place. Chicory ranks so highly because of its versatility and ease of use; lamb's lettuce has a lovely thick, dense texture that soothes the appetite. Now it is available ready-prepared in packets, its sole drawback has disappeared – previously it had to be carefully washed to remove any sand. Lamb's lettuce has a very mild flavour and, in fact, it has an alternative name in French, *doucette*, which means mild. Although it is gentle in taste, its thick, dense texture will satisfy your appetite. You can easily grow it in your back garden, but when preparing it do make sure you remove any sand, which remains its one main downside.

How to prepare and eat lamb's lettuce in the Dukan Diet

Lamb's lettuce is eaten raw in salads; beetroot is its best partner as both vegetables have great sweetness. Do not swamp the mild, delicate flavour of your lamb's lettuce by combining it with strong-tasting or highly-flavoured vegetables and dressings.

Lamb's lettuce and smoked salmon rolls

Ballotins de mâche au saumon fumé

100g (3½oz) fat-free fromage
  frais
Handful of chopped fresh
  chives, plus a few whole
  chives for tying
Juice of 2 lemons
Salt and black pepper
4 slices smoked salmon
1 bunch of lamb's lettuce

Phase 2 PV

Preparation time: 10 minutes
2 servings

Make a dressing with the fromage frais, chopped chives and a quarter of the lemon juice. Add a little salt.

Lay out the slices of smoked salmon and spread the lamb's lettuce over them. Divide the dressing equally between the 4 salmon slices, then roll them up and tie them together with the whole chives to keep them in place. Pour over the remaining lemon juice.

89. Leek

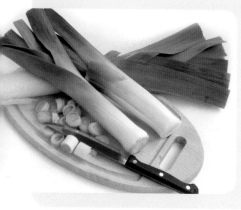

Leeks are not a great favourite with children and tend to be a vegetable that adults gradually come to enjoy. In France their use is quite specific and limited to the traditional leek vinaigrette salad and to being an ingredient in stews. The best bit of a leek, and often the only part that is eaten, is the 'white part'.

General nutritional characteristics

As far as nutrition goes, leeks have an average number of calories (21 per 100g). Their great plus point is that they are diuretic, making them even more of a must-eat for women who suffer from water retention.

Role in the Dukan Diet

If you choose your leeks carefully and cook them correctly, the white part of the leek does not deserve to be regarded as the 'poor man's asparagus'. When you are losing weight, leeks have much more to offer as a vegetable than asparagus as they are denser, tastier and more satisfying.

How to prepare and eat leek in the Dukan Diet

I wholeheartedly recommend using them as an accompanying vegetable, finished off in a wok or frying pan, after having been steamed first. If you cook them gently for a long time they develop a caramelized taste that can add a lot of flavour to your cooking. After they have been cooked, you can also use a blender to mix them with some eggs, oat bran and fromage frais to make a gratin dish, finished off with a dusting of Parmesan cheese on top.

Leek and ham quiche
Quiche jambon-poireaux

3 leeks sliced
Salt and black pepper
5 eggs
10 tablespoons fat-free
  fromage frais
3 slices rind-free, fat-free
  pre-cooked ham or turkey,
  cut into thin strips

For the Dukan galette base
2 tablespoons wheat bran
4 tablespoons oat bran
4 tablespoons fromage frais
2 egg whites

Phase 2 PV

Preparation time: 15 minutes
Cooking time: 20 minutes
2 servings

Preheat the oven to 180°C/350°F/Gas 4.

Mix together the galette ingredients and pour into a flan dish lined with greaseproof paper. Bake in the oven for about 12 minutes, then remove and set aside.

Soften the leeks in a frying pan with a little water. Season with salt and black pepper. In a bowl, whisk together the eggs and fromage frais. Add the strips of sliced meat and season to taste.

Arrange the leeks on top of the galette, then pour over the egg, ham and fromage frais mixture. Bake in the oven for about 20 minutes until set and golden on top.

90. Lettuce

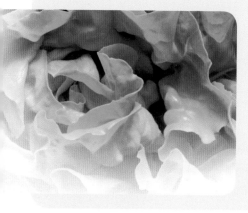

Lettuce is the salad ingredient _par excellence_ and a great ally when you are losing weight. Along with tomatoes, lettuce is the favourite vegetable in France, where it is customarily eaten with a vinaigrette dressing.

General nutritional characteristics
Extremely low in calories (between 8 and 11 per 100g depending on the variety), lettuce does, however, soak up oil when it is dressed, so you need to use our Dukan vinaigrette dressing (see page 223) instead. Lettuce offers a good range of different vitamins, minerals and trace elements.

Role in the Dukan Diet
Lettuce has the advantage in my diet of providing the taste of salad leaves with the hint of something sweet, which is always welcome in a programme heavily weighted towards proteins. In Europe, the young round lettuce is most widely used as it is the most tender variety and has the whitest lettuce heart. Frisée or curly endive is crunchier, but it guzzles up dressing. Some lettuce varieties have a slight nutty flavour. Cos lettuce is firmer and more brittle.

How to prepare and eat lettuce in the Dukan Diet
Lettuce can be braised or put into soups but I would not recommend this as it loses its crunch, its lovely green colour and some of its vitamins – folic acid in particular, which is so important for women.

Spring lettuce rolls
Rouleaux de laitue printaniers

150g (5½oz) fat-free natural yoghurt
1 tablespoon lemon juice
1 teaspoon chopped fresh chives
1 tablespoon chopped fresh mint
Salt and black pepper
1 small cucumber

200g (7oz) cooked prawns, shelled
100g (3½oz) soya bean sprouts
100g (3½oz) fat-free fromage frais
4 large lettuce leaves

Phase 2 PV

Preparation time: 20 minutes
4 servings

In a bowl, mix together the yoghurt, lemon juice, chives and mint. Season with salt and black pepper and refrigerate.

Remove four long strips from the cucumber skin using a vegetable peeler and cut them in half; set aside. Grate the cucumber and place in a sieve with a little salt to make it disgorge its water. Once the water has drained off, combine the cucumber with the prawns, soya bean sprouts and fromage frais. Season with salt and black pepper.

Spread this mixture over the lettuce leaves and roll them up. Using scissors, trim the edges of the lettuce so that they are even, then tie the rolls up with the reserved strips of cucumber skin. Serve the rolls on plates with some of the yoghurt dressing spooned over.

91. Mushrooms

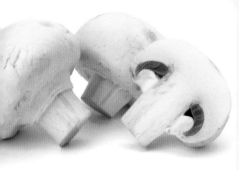

Halfway between animal and vegetable, mushrooms are often seen as a sort of vegetable 'meat' because of their firm, resistant texture. The most common representative of the mushroom family is the button mushroom, as it is grown on an industrial scale. Wild mushrooms are a luxury food item for occasional pleasure.

General nutritional characteristics

As far as nutrition goes, the button mushroom is a pseudo-vegetable. It is low in calories (35 per 100g), with almost 3g proteins per 100g.

Role in the Dukan Diet

In my diet, what makes mushrooms so prized is precisely their unusual texture and their ability to make us feel full up. Moreover, they contain more protein than most green vegetables. Mushrooms are a vegetable that, as a rule, almost everyone enjoys; they also help to introduce some diversity into the diet as they are the only vegetable that can survive without chlorophyll.

How to prepare and eat mushrooms in the Dukan Diet

The button mushroom can be eaten cooked or raw. Raw, it makes a good salad ingredient. If you come across a really big mushroom, slice it very finely, from top to bottom including the stalk, arrange it on a nice plate and tap it so that the slices spread out into a fan shape. Then add some sauce – for example, a little Dukan vinaigrette dressing (see page 223) – using a spray. Cook button mushrooms by frying them lightly in a pan (with three drops of oil wiped using kitchen paper), or stuff them with a meat or salmon tartare filling. They are also great with omelettes, either as an accompaniment or as an ingredient chopped up with some finely cut ham, and they can be added in the same way to oat bran galettes. So that you never run out, always keep a bag of mushrooms in your freezer! There are also other types of mushrooms that go particularly well with meat and poultry.

Creamy button mushrooms
Crème de champignons de Paris

500g (1lb 2oz) button
  mushrooms
1 bunch fresh tarragon
4 slices bresaola
250ml (9fl oz) 3% fat crème
  fraîche
Salt and black pepper

Phase 2 PV

Preparation time: 15 minutes +
  1 hour resting
Cooking time: 10 minutes
6 servings

Wash and chop the mushrooms and tarragon, reserving a few whole tarragon leaves to use as a garnish. Roughly chop the bresaola. Gently fry the mushrooms with the bresaola and tarragon.

Blend the mushroom mixture with the crème fraîche and season with salt and black pepper. Pour the mushroom cream into individual dishes and leave to rest for at least 1 hour before serving with the reserved tarragon leaves sprinkled over.

92. Onion

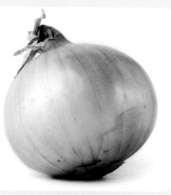

When it comes to cooking, losing weight and keeping healthy, onions are one of the most precious foods-condiments we have.

General nutritional characteristics

Nutritionally, for 31 calories per 100g, 8g of carbohydrates and 0g fat, you get a medicinal food that should be sold in your local pharmacy. Onions provide the best vegetable source of selenium, which really boosts the power of vitamin E. They contain plenty of vitamins E and C, and combine the big players in cardiovascular protection as they also help to fluidify the blood, which reduces its tendency to clot. Being rich in sulphur, onions prevent glucose levels in the blood from rising and thus offer protection against diabetes. Lastly, they contain rare substances such as manganese, cobalt, fluorine and molybdenum.

Role in the Dukan Diet

Onions are so completely unavoidable in my diet that I would ask anyone who dislikes them to come up with an 'attachment' strategy. In France, it is difficult for a cook to work without using any garlic, onions, salt or pepper. Once cooked enough to get rid of the sulphur compounds (they sting, make you cry and make your breath smelly), onions turn out to be mild and even sweet with a caramelized flavour. They also have diuretic properties that are slight but sufficient to help any women suffering from water retention.

How to prepare and eat onion in the Dukan Diet

Onions can be used equally well raw or cooked, mild or spicy, in salads, in main dishes as an accompaniment and even in puddings. Think of Chinese beef with onions or Spanish onion tortillas; then there is the vast array of Mediterranean dishes that use onions extensively and, in France, the many '*à la soubise*' recipes which include onion purée. Onions can be also be baked in the oven and may even be stuffed.

Onion sauce
Sauce à l'oignon

1 large onion, finely chopped
1 small glass vegetable stock
1 egg yolk
15g (½oz) virtually fat-free
  quark
15g (½oz) fat-free fromage
  frais
1 teaspoon balsamic vinegar

1 teaspoon mustard
Salt and black pepper

Phase 1 PP / Phase 2 PP

Preparation time: 5 minutes
Cooking time: 2 minutes
2 servings

In a pan, gently cook the onion in the stock for 2 minutes, then set aside to cool.

In a bowl, combine the egg yolk, quark, fromage frais, vinegar, mustard, salt and black pepper. Very gradually stir in the cooled onion mixture and make sure everything is well mixed together. Serve cold.

93. Palm hearts

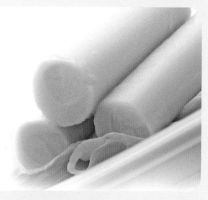

The heart of palm is the final bud of a tree, the palm tree. This is a wild, forest product, not cultivated by man and not grown intensively. Once tinned it becomes a very useful vegetable and for this reason appears among my 100 foods. Select a top-quality product to ensure that your palm hearts are tender and not stringy.

General nutritional characteristics

As far as nutrition goes, palm hearts contain only 25 calories per 100g with 2.3g protein.

Role in the Dukan Diet

Because of their firm, resistant texture palm hearts make you chew really hard. They are low in calories and for a plant they contain a lot of protein. They are unusual, exotic and offer a little variety. Lastly, as they come in a tin or jar ready to use straightaway, they are a practical option in my diet.

How to prepare and eat palm hearts in the Dukan Diet

Use them like a vegetable, either in a mixed salad or as a support act, but always eat them with a Dukan vinaigrette dressing (see page 223). Cooked, they work as an accompaniment or garnish equally well with poultry, meat and fish dishes. If you are eating them this way, try them with a Dukan béchamel sauce (see page 222) or some homemade tomato sauce. My favourite recipe is palm hearts rolled up in smoked salmon with lemon and dill.

Smoked salmon and palm heart rolls

Roulés de saumon fumé aux cœurs de palmier

6 palm hearts
6 slices smoked salmon
250g (9oz) virtually fat-free
  quark
1 garlic clove, crushed
Handful of chopped fresh
  herbs
150ml (5fl oz) skimmed milk

Pinch of curry powder
Salt and black pepper

Phase 2 PV

Preparation time: 10 minutes
6 servings

Roll up each palm heart in a slice of smoked salmon and put them in the fridge.

Mix together the quark, garlic and herbs with the skimmed milk and add the curry powder. If necessary, season to taste with salt and black pepper, and add a little more milk if the cream is too thick.

Serve the chilled palm heart rolls on plates with the sauce poured over.

94. Peppers

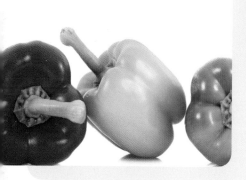

A vegetable-fruit with extremely dense flesh and a crisp, crunchy texture as well as a sweet taste (red variety only), peppers are juicy, clean, easy to carry around and can be eaten in many different ways.

General nutritional characteristics
Peppers are, along with cabbage, the vegetables with the most vitamin C (they contain even more than oranges). They are also rich in vitamin A, potassium and folic acid, and you get all this for just 27 calories per 100g.

Role in the Dukan Diet
Peppers are a leading player in my diet. Raw, they go into salads along with tomatoes: for example, in a *salade niçoise*. They can also be eaten just as they are with dips or cut into strips. Cooked, they make a great stuffed vegetable as they can hold a lot and keep their shape in the oven.

How to prepare and eat peppers in the Dukan Diet
A marvellous way of preparing them is 'grilled': pop them in the oven and keep turning them over until the skin goes black. Then leave them in a small, airtight plastic bag until they have cooled down; the skin will come off easily. At this point you have two options, the princely and the imperial. The princely option is to cut them into strips, add roughly chopped garlic, salt and pepper, and then wait. A thick juice will appear that will make you think your peppers are swimming in oil – a mirage for your eyes and taste buds. The imperial option is only for summer when the sun is strong. Place some whole peppers on a wooden slab and leave them out all day in the sun. The next day turn them over until they have dried out and the skin has gone leathery. Then put them in a jar with some flavoured oil, salt, pepper and paprika and leave for at least 45 days before you eat them, but do wipe them beforehand with some kitchen paper. Have you ever felt before that you were 'eating sunshine'?

Three-pepper chicken
Poulet aux trois poivrons

1 red pepper
1 yellow pepper
1 green pepper
4 very thin chicken breasts
Salt and black pepper
Handful of fresh thyme
Juice of 2 lemons

Phase 2 PV

Preparation time: 10 minutes +
  1 hour marinating
Cooking time: 10 minutes
4 servings

Wash the peppers and cut them into very thin strips. Cut the chicken breasts in two lengthways. Season them with salt and black pepper and sprinkle over the fresh thyme.

Make up little bundles of the pepper strips and lay them across each piece of meat. Roll up each breast and use a wooden cocktail stick to keep the chicken rolls in place and make mini kebabs. Season with a little of the lemon juice and refrigerate for 1 hour.

Prepare a grill pan or your barbecue and remove the chicken from the fridge. Cook your mini kebabs for 8–10 minutes, turning them round halfway through.

Serve with some more of the lemon juice squeezed over.

95. Pumpkin

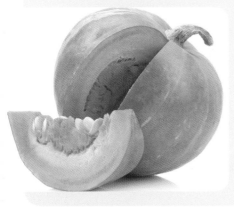

Pumpkins are exceptional vegetables because of their size, colour and texture, their sweetness and biological value…and let's not forget that magical pumpkin soup!

General nutritional characteristics

Pumpkin contains few calories (26 per 100g), and 5g carbohydrates per 100g, but it is very rich in vitamin A (a 200g/7oz portion provides a man's daily requirement).

Role in the Dukan Diet

Pumpkin is full of pectin, the same pectin that we find in apples, with many of its medicinal qualities. But what really interests us is that pectin traps calories in the stomach and then eliminates them from the body in our stools. Eating pumpkin means you lose calories, so for dieters this vegetable is a true friend. In addition, pumpkin has an appealing colour and a sweetness that is most welcome to anyone feeling bereft of sugary foods to snack on. A nice slice of firm pumpkin, steamed, served with some vanilla or cinnamon sprinkled on top, can distract you from such cravings.

How to prepare and eat pumpkin in the Dukan Diet

Traditionally, pumpkin is made into soup or mash, which children love because of Halloween – as well as for the taste. Once they grow up, these children will invariably remain pumpkin fans. So one evening when it is really cold outside, make yourself some pumpkin soup and add a tablespoon of low-fat crème fraîche; it will warm you up immediately and bring you comfort so that you feel at peace with the world. Personally, I have a weakness for thick slices of pumpkin, steamed but still *al dente* so that they keep their shape without collapsing, over which I trickle a little soy sauce – this is so delicious, you just have to try it!

Pumpkin loaf
Cake au potiron

400g (14oz) pumpkin flesh, cut into 1cm (½in) cubes	50g (1¾oz) oat bran	**Phase 2 PV**
3 eggs	1 teaspoon baking powder	**Preparation time: 15 minutes**
10 drops melted butter flavouring (www.mydukandietshop.co.uk)	150g (5½oz) cooked chicken, cut into sticks	**Cooking time: 65 minutes**
20 drops chestnut flavouring (www.mydukandietshop.co.uk)	100g (3½oz) Emmental or other hard cheese (5% fat) (tolerated)	**8 servings**
100ml (3½fl oz) skimmed milk	A little chopped fresh parsley	
50g (1¾oz) wholemeal flour	A little grated nutmeg	
	Salt and black pepper	

Cook the pumpkin in a non-stick frying pan along with 4 tablespoons water. Stir from time to time and add more water if necessary. After about 15 minutes, use the tip of a knife to check whether it is cooked. If the knife goes in easily, remove the pan from the heat. Purée in a blender, then put to one side.

Preheat the oven to 220°C/425°F/Gas 7.

In a bowl, whisk the eggs with the flavourings to produce an omelette mixture. Then add the pumpkin purée, milk, flour, oat bran and baking powder. Stir together well. Fold in the chicken sticks and cheese. Add some parsley, nutmeg, salt and black pepper.

Pour the mixture into a loaf tin or a soufflé mould and bake in the oven for 50 minutes. Check to see whether the loaf is cooked by inserting the tip of a knife – it should come out clean.

96. Radish

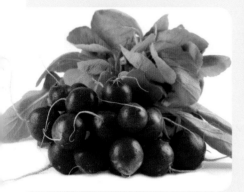

Radishes are a great little vegetable for losing weight. They could almost be an appetizer, a bite-size *amuse-gueule*, when not used in a starter. Black winter radishes, which taste very hot, have their admirers too.

General nutritional characteristics

Radishes are low in calories (20 per 100g) and, as with most vegetables, a good source of vitamin C, potassium and folic acid.

Role in the Dukan Diet

Only ever eaten raw, radishes are fresh, firm, crunchy, requiring nothing but a little salt. Colourful and easy to carry around, they are handy for people who take a lunchbox to work. Their only drawback, which can be a problem nowadays, is that they have to be washed and prepared. Their tops and root ends need to be chopped off, and sometimes a bit of the skin – which gives them their distinct spicy flavour – needs to be peeled too.

How to prepare and eat radish in the Dukan Diet

Sprinkle on a little salt and nothing else – then enjoy!

Eggs stuffed with quark and black winter radish

Œufs farcis au carré frais 0% et au radis noir

6 eggs
50g (1¾oz) black winter
  radish, grated
100g (3½oz) virtually fat-free
  quark
Salt and black pepper

Phase 2 PV

Preparation time: 10 minutes
Cooking time: 10 minutes
6 servings

Boil the eggs for about 10 minutes, then run under cold water for a minute or two. When they are cool enough to handle, shell the hard-boiled eggs, rinse and drain.

Cut the eggs in half and remove the yolks without damaging the whites. Put the quark, radish and yolks in a bowl and season with salt and black pepper. Combine the ingredients thoroughly to obtain a smooth mixture. Taste and adjust the seasoning.

Using a small spoon, fill each egg-white half with the radish mixture and serve.

97. Rhubarb

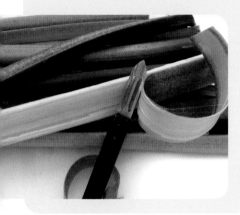

Rhubarb is a food that is not always that highly regarded because of its laxative qualities, the uncertainty as to whether it is actually a fruit or a vegetable, and the fact that it needs to be cooked before it can be eaten.

General nutritional characteristics

At 15 calories per 100g and only 2g carbohydrates, rhubarb is an absolute marvel. It is a good source of vitamin C (12mg per 100g) and magnesium, good for relaxation and energy. Do be careful, though, as the effect it has on bowel movements means that people who suffer from colitis or who have a sensitive stomach should avoid eating it. Lastly, being rich in oxalic acid, it is not recommended for anyone with stones in their urinary tract.

Role in the Dukan Diet

Rhubarb is ranked as a master food in my diet as it is the only fruit allowed during the Attack and Cruise phases, which get you down to your True Weight. It allows you the only opportunity there is in these two phases for making jams and fruit compote, which are otherwise banned. Along with the oat bran galette, another master food, it allows you to make tartlets, muffins, creams and mousses! To do this, you will have to add some sweetener, Aspartame or polyols (sugar-free sweeteners), to hide the rhubarb's natural acidity. Another advantage of rhubarb is that it improves bowel regularity, thereby helping to remedy one of the usual drawbacks of my fat-free diet, the slowing down of stool movements. Lastly, it is hard to find a food with fewer calories and with so little carbohydrate, especially given that it tastes like a fruit.

How to prepare and eat rhubarb in the Dukan Diet

To stew rhubarb, cook the stalks in a little water for 20 minutes to soften, but do not overcook or it will turn into a mush. Then add sweetener. Rhubarb teams well with cinnamon, lemon and ginger. It can also be used in savoury dishes as an accompaniment to meat or fish.

Rhubarb clafoutis
Clafoutis de rhubarbe

4 eggs
8 tablespoons powdered
  sweetener, or more
  according to taste
20g (¾oz) cornflour
400ml (14fl oz) skimmed milk
600g (1lb 5oz) rhubarb, fresh
  or frozen

Phase 2 PV

Preparation time: 10 minutes
Cooking time: 40 minutes
4 servings

Preheat the oven to 180°C/350°F/Gas 4.

Whisk the eggs into an omelette mixture with the sweetener. Dissolve the cornflour in a little of the cold milk, then pour it into the eggs and add the rest of the milk.

Cut the rhubarb into small chunks and arrange them in a non-stick dish. Pour the egg mixture over the rhubarb and bake in a bain-marie in the oven for 40 minutes.

98. Soya bean sprouts

Soya bean sprouts are a great vegetable for slimming. However, do be careful: soya can mean a bean and therefore a legume when the seed has not germinated; it becomes a vegetable only after germination and after the sprout has developed, using up the seed's store of fats and carbohydrates.

General nutritional characteristics

Soya bean sprouts have more calories than most vegetables (57 per 100g); they are also a medicinal vegetable. As the vegetable containing the most top-quality proteins, soya bean sprouts almost rival meat. They also contain phytoestrogens, exactly what menopausal women need.

Role in the Dukan Diet

As far as helping with slimming is concerned, you must go for fresh soya beans picked very young before they turn oily and starchy, i.e. with fats and sugar. At this stage, the young bean is very rich in proteins and very filling, with a nice, nutty flavour and dense texture. It makes an excellent contribution to the Dukan Diet. When soya is more mature, dried or turned into soya flour, it then appears in the diet only during the Consolidation phase.

How to prepare and eat soya bean sprouts in the Dukan Diet

Soya bean sprouts can be eaten cooked – for example, in Chinese chop suey – or raw in Vietnamese or Thai salads, along with strips of cooked chicken or prawns and crab, with a tasty dressing made from wine vinegar and soy sauce. They are one of the main ingredients in spring rolls.

Chinese chicken bites with soya bean sprouts

Bouchées de poulet et soja à la chinoise

300g (10½oz) chicken breast, cubed
Soya bean sprouts

For the marinade
Juice of 2 lemons
3 tablespoons soy sauce
1 tablespoon mustard
Salt and black pepper

Phase 2 PV

Preparation time: 40 minutes +
1 hour marinating
Cooking time: 15 minutes
2 servings

Prepare the marinade. Pour the lemon juice, soy sauce and mustard into a medium-sized bowl, and season with salt and black pepper. Add the chicken and mix all the ingredients together. Cover with clingfilm and refrigerate for at least 1 hour, stirring from time to time.

Warm the grill or the barbecue. Remove the chicken from the fridge and retain the marinade. Cook the chicken for about 7 minutes, then turn the meat over, baste with a little of the marinade and cook for a further 7 minutes.

Meanwhile, heat a few spoonfuls of the remaining marinade in a frying pan with the soya bean sprouts. Fry them for about 10 minutes and serve with the chicken bites.

99. Spinach

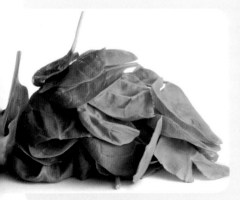

Nowadays, spinach tends to be eaten cooked rather than raw, from tins rather than prepared from scratch, and from frozen in preference to tinned. It is not everybody's favourite vegetable; there are few children who clamour for it. However, the enjoyment of spinach often depends on how it is cooked.

General nutritional characteristics

Very low in calories (18 per 100g), spinach is a great source of folic acid, essential for pregnant women and people with heart problems. It is well known for containing lots of iron (as symbolized by Popeye's biceps) and for its high vitamin A content. This is a healthy vegetable but you have to like it and to do that you have to know how to cook it.

Role in the Dukan Diet

In my method and diet, which is mostly followed by women, spinach is an invaluable vegetable because of its iron, which women are so often lacking if they have heavy periods or menstrual cycles that come too close together. It is recommended that you prepare it with meat juices, which are also full of iron, or with some stock. A simpler way is to prepare it by adding some extra-light cream (3–4% fat).

How to prepare and eat spinach in the Dukan Diet

Spinach goes really well with milk, fromage frais and eggs (mixed into omelettes or as a gratin baked in the oven with a little Parmesan dusting on top). It can also be used as an ingredient in stuffing. Spinach makes a good vegetable accompaniment for veal, poultry and fish, particularly salmon where the colour combination looks really attractive.

Scallop and spinach clafoutis
Clafoutis de Saint-Jacques aux épinards

300g (10½oz) frozen scallops,
  thawed
Salt and black pepper
250g (9oz) frozen spinach,
  thawed
1 egg plus 1 egg white
30g (1oz) cornflour
125ml (4fl oz) skimmed milk
2 tablespoons silken tofu

Phase 2 PV

Preparation time: 20 minutes
Cooking time: 25 minutes
4 servings

Preheat the oven to 180°C/350°F/Gas 4.

Dry the scallops and season them with some salt and black pepper.
Gently fry the scallops in a frying pan lightly oiled and wiped with
kitchen paper.

Heat the spinach in a pan for 5 minutes, then squeeze out the water.

Whisk together the whole egg and the egg white with the cornflour.
Blend with the milk and silken tofu. Season with salt and black pepper.

Spread the spinach over the bottom of an ovenproof dish and arrange
the scallops on top. Pour over the tofu mixture and bake in the oven for
about 25 minutes.

100. Tomato

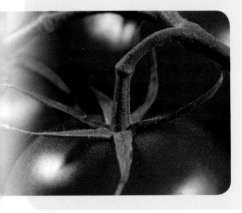

In the Dukan Diet, the tomato is one of the most essential vegetables and one of the foods most representative of our universal diet. Thanks to modern transport methods, we are able to buy them all year round.

General nutritional characteristics

Very low in calories (20 per 100g), tomatoes are rich in vitamins B, K and C and in lycopene (the pigment that gives them their colour and which is very similar to carotene).

Role in the Dukan Diet

Simply enjoying tomatoes and eating them regularly is of enormous help in fighting weight problems. Conversely, not eating them makes it easier to put weight on. The reason why tomatoes are so useful is that they can be used in so many ways, raw in salads, or just as they are with a little salt or vinaigrette dressing. They are easy to take around with you because of their firm skin. They have a slightly acidic flavour and are very juicy, which means you can eat them without any dressing at all (i.e. without any oil) – just cut them up and sprinkle over a little salt.

How to prepare and eat tomato in the Dukan Diet

Cooked, tomatoes can be stuffed Provence-style with mince and herbs. They are a key ingredient in ratatouille, gazpacho and, of course, tomato sauce. They team up well with garlic, shallots, basil, tarragon, thyme, bay leaves, oregano and cumin (and do remember that the more you flavour your food, the more weight you will lose and the more easily too). Tomatoes also complement fish proteins brilliantly, such as tuna, sardines and mullet, and the same goes for meat – beef, chicken, veal – and eggs. You can buy tinned tomatoes with different sauces, chopped, or as passata or purée. You can even drink tomato juice as an aperitif. When dried, tomatoes develop an exquisite flavour – just blot with kitchen paper to remove the oil.

Stuffed beef tomatoes
Tomates coeur de boeuf farcies

2 onions, finely chopped
2 garlic cloves, finely chopped
1 shallot, finely chopped
250g (8oz) minced beefsteak
   (5% fat)
Handful of chopped fresh
   parsley
Salt and black pepper
4 large beef tomatoes

Phase 2 PV

Preparation time: 10 minutes
Cooking time: 45 minutes
2 servings

Preheat the oven to 180°C/350°F/Gas 4.

Place the onions, garlic and shallot in a non-stick frying pan with
3 tablespoons water. Once the frying pan is properly hot, remove it from
the heat and add the minced beef, parsley, salt and black pepper.

Cut a lid off each tomato about 1cm (½in) from the top, scoop out the
seeds and remove all the juice. Remove all the tomato flesh and add to
the meat stuffing mixture.

Fill the tomatoes with the stuffing mixture and bake in the oven for
45 minutes.

Dukan béchamel sauce
La béchamel Dukan

100ml (3½fl oz) skimmed milk
2 tablespoons cornflour
Black pepper
Pinch of grated nutmeg (optional)

In a pan, combine the cold skimmed milk with the cornflour. Cook the mixture over a low heat for a few minutes, stirring continually as the sauce thickens, then season with some black pepper and a pinch of nutmeg (if using).

Dukan mayonnaise
La mayonnaise Dukan

3 egg yolks, at room temperature
1 teaspoon vinegar
Pinch of salt
Pinch of chopped fresh parsley
 (optional)
2 teaspoons mustard
75ml (2½fl oz) olive oil

Put the egg yolks in a small, deep bowl and add the vinegar, salt, parsley (if using) and mustard. Let the mixture rest for 5 minutes without touching it, then stir the ingredients together very carefully using a teaspoon.

Using a hand-held blender – check first that it touches the bottom of your bowl – blend the mixture. Start off using circular movements while adding small drizzles of olive oil.

After 1 minute, increase the speed of the blender and move it from top to bottom while continuing to drizzle in the remainder of the oil very gradually. Make sure that the blade of the blender always remains in contact with the mixture and carry on blending until your mayonnaise is quite firm and white.

Dukan vinaigrette dressing
La vinaigrette Dukan

½ tablespoon mustard
Pinch of salt
Black pepper
2 tablespoons balsamic (or other) vinegar
2 tablespoons olive oil
2 tablespoons Perrier water

In a bowl, mix together the mustard, salt, some black pepper and the balsamic vinegar until you get a smooth sauce.

Add the olive oil and Perrier water, then use a fork to stir up the sauce.

First published in France in 2010 by Éditions J'ai lu

First published in Great Britain in 2012 by Hodder & Stoughton
An Hachette UK company

1

A CIP catalogue record for this title is available from the British Library

Trade Paperback ISBN 978 1 444 75786 6
Ebook ISBN 978 1 444 75787 3

Translated by Morag Jordan

Designed by Bobby&Co

Typeset in Helvetica Std and ITC Flora

Printed and bound in Spain by Gráficas Estella

Hodder & Stoughton policy is to use papers that are natural, renewable and recyclable products and made from wood grown in sustainable forests. The logging and manufacturing processes are expected to conform to the environmental regulations of the country of origin.

Hodder & Stoughton Ltd
338 Euston Road
London NW1 3BH

www.hodder.co.uk